EDUCATION AND HIV/AIDS
IN THE CARIBBEAN

EDUCATION AND HIV/AIDS
IN THE CARIBBEAN

Michael J. Kelly

Brendan Bain

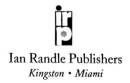

Ian Randle Publishers
Kingston • Miami

UNESCO Office
for the Caribbean

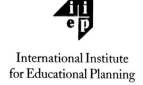

International Institute
for Educational Planning

3 04211

JUN 1 0 2005

Original title: *Education and HIV/AIDS in the Caribbean*
by Michael J. Kelly

First published by the United Nations Educational, Scientific and Cultural
Organization: International Institute for Educational Planning (UNESCO-IIEP)
7-9 rue Eugène - Delacroix
75116 Paris, France

Published 2005, by
Ian Randle Publishers
11 Cunningham Avenue
Box 686
Kingston 6
www.ianrandlepublishers.com

National Library of Jamaica Cataloguing in Publication Data

Kelly, Michael J.
    Education and HIV/AIDS in the Caribbean / Michael J. Kelly, Brendan Bain

        p. : ill., maps ;   cm.

    Includes index

    ISBN 976-637-180-6 (pbk)

    1. AIDS (Disease) – Caribbean Area - Prevention   2. AIDS (Disease) – Caribbean
    Area – Study and teaching   3. HIV infections – Caribbean Area   4. Health
    education – Caribbean Area
    I. Bain, Brendan   II. Title

    614.599392   dc 21

Cover image courtesy of the Jamaica AIDS Support Anti-Stigma and Discrimination
Campaign, 2004. Photography: Jeremy Francis; Make-up: Cecile Burrowes, Jeni
Francis; Art Direction: Pierre Lemaire.

Cover and book design by Allison Brown
Printed in the USA

CONTENTS

ILLUSTRATIONS

Boxes

Figures

Tables

ABBREVIATIONS

ACU	Association of Commonwealth Universities
AIDS	Acquired Immunodeficiency Syndrome
CAPNET	Caribbean Publishers Network
CAREC	Caribbean Epidemiology Centre
CARICOM	Caribbean Community
CARNA	Caribbean Red Cross Network on AIDS
CCM	Country Coordinating Mechanism
CDC	Centre for Disease Control and Prevention
CGCED	Caribbean Group for Cooperation in Economic Development
CHRC	Caribbean Health Research Council
CIDA	Canadian International Development Agency
CRC	Convention on the Rights of the Child
CRN+	Caribbean Network of People Living with HIV/AIDS
CRSPAH	Caribbean Regional Strategic Plan of Action for HIV/AIDS
DFID	Department for International Development
EFA	Education for All
EI	Education International
EIC	Excitement, Involvement, Commitment
EMIS	Education Management Information System
EU	European Union
FBO	Faith-Based Organisation
FRESH	Focusing Resources on Effective School Health
GDP	Gross Domestic Product
GFATM	Global Fund to Fight AIDS, Tuberculosis and Malaria
GNI	Gross National Income
HARP	HIV/AIDS Response Programme
HDI	Human Development Index
HEARD	Health Economics and AIDS Research Division
HFLE	Health and Family Life Education
HIV	Human Immuno-deficiency Virus
HPV	Human Papilloma Virus
IAEN	International AIDS Economics Network
IATT	Inter-Agency Task Team
IBE	International Bureau of Education
ICASA	International Conference on AIDS and Sexually Transmitted Diseases in Africa

IEC	Information, Education and Communication
IIEP	International Institute for Educational Planning
ILO	International Labour Organization
IT	Information Technology
KABP	Knowledge, Attitudes, Beliefs and Practices
MENJS	Ministère de l'Éducation nationale, de la Jeunesse et des Sports
MOE	Ministry of Education
NAP	National AIDS Programme
NCC	Non-Campus Country
NGO	Non-Governmental Organization
OECS	Organization of Eastern Caribbean States
PAHO	Pan-American Health Organization
PANCAP	Pan-Caribbean Partnership Against HIV/AIDS
PLA	Person Living with HIV/AIDS
PTCT	Parent to Child Transmission
SIRHASC	Strengthening the Institutional Response to HIV/AIDS/STIs in the Caribbean
SMART	Specific, Measurable, Achievable, Realistic and Timebound
SRH	Sexual and Reproductive Health
STD	Sexually Transmitted Disease
STI	Sexually Transmitted Infection
SWOT	Strengths, Weaknesses, Opportunities, Threats
TB	Tuberculosis
TV	Television
UN	United Nations
UNAIDS	Joint United Nations Programme on HIV/AIDS
UNDCP	United Nations Drug Control Programme
UNDP	United Nations Development Programme
UNECA	United Nations Economic Commission for Africa
UNESCO	United Nations Educational, Scientific and Cultural Organization
UNFPA	United Nations Population Fund
UNGASS	United Nations General Assembly Special Session
UNICA	Association of Caribbean Universities and Research Institutes
UNICEF	United Nations Children's Fund
UNIFEM	United Nations Development Fund for Women
US	United States
USAID	United States Agency for International Development
UWI	The University of the West Indies
UWI HARP	The University of the West Indies HIV/AIDS Response Programme
VCT	Voluntary Counselling and Testing
WHO	World Health Organization

FOREWORD

I would like to express my sincere gratitude on behalf of UNESCO and the International Institute of Educational Planning, and on behalf of our member states in the Caribbean, to Michael Kelly, Brendan Bain and Rex Nettleford, who undertook just one year ago to jointly develop a strategic framework to guide the response of education in the region to this devastating epidemic. This seminal work is the result.

Its publication is most timely. The Ministers of Education of Caribbean countries jointly endorsed the need for such a strategy when UNESCO hosted them in Havana in November 2002. For Governments and leaders of Caribbean society, it is a 'wake-up' call on the critical role of education – both formal and non-formal – as multisectoral responses to HIV/AIDS are being fashioned. The book makes a strong case for an equal role of education, alongside health and other sectors, if the scourge of AIDS is to be effectively tackled. UNESCO has brought together African and Caribbean expertise and experience to create this new valuable tool in the struggle against HIV/AIDS.

Even as this strategy was being drafted, it was informing the thinking of UNESCO in the Caribbean, and we have not waited on the launch of the publication to act. Several partnerships have already been established and capacity-building activities are underway – for education officials, media leaders, educational publishers, teacher educators and HIV/AIDS coordinators in education ministries. UNESCO in the Caribbean now works in partnership with several regional organizations, development banks and donors to this end. Readers wishing to find out more about how UNESCO has been contributing to the actualization of the strategy resented in this book, can visit our web site at www.unescocaribbean.org and click on Education: HIV/AIDS, or write directly to me at kingston@unesco.org. Our quarterly electronic report on Education and AIDS is available to all who are interested.

We recognize that this strategy is merely a road map, but without such a map effective action is impossible to visualize and plan. UNESCO is hopeful that it will provide the impetus for even greater cooperation among all concerned in the Caribbean to bring the full potential of the education sector to bear on the most critical and challenging of problems, AIDS.

Lastly, I would like to thank Michael Morrissey, an international expert on education and my able consultant here at the UNESCO's Office for the Caribbean for the past year, without whose support and dedication this book would not have been published.

Hélène-Marie Gosselin
Director, UNESCO Office for the Caribbean

PREFACE AND ACKNOWLEDGEMENTS

This book is addressed to those who are concerned about the interaction between the HIV/AIDS epidemic and the education sector in Caribbean countries. One of its recurrent themes is that education's response to the epidemic will depend heavily on the combined efforts of a wide range of partners. These include education policy-makers, managers and administrators, institutional heads and their senior staff, parents and community leaders, those in non-governmental and faith-based organisations that work in the field of education, youth leaders and media personnel, personnel from health and other relevant public sectors, youth leaders and role models, persons living with HIV/AIDS, and those in education-related areas in bilateral and multilateral agencies.

The book evolved out of a desire to equip all of these with information and understanding on what the epidemic means, or could mean, for educational provision in the region, and on the diverse ways education contributes, or could contribute, to managing HIV/AIDS, slowing down its further spread, and eventually rolling it back. The authors hope that the volume will strengthen the commitment of its readers in their efforts to minimise the impact of the AIDS epidemic on the education sector and maximise the impact of education on the epidemic.

We are grateful to the many people who have supported the development and production of this book. Special thanks go to the International Institute for Educational Planning in Paris and UNESCO's Office for the Caribbean for commissioning us as authors and for the financial support that made it possible for us to work together. The energetic and resourceful leadership shown on both sides of the

Atlantic in promoting this work gives clear expression to the dynamic role UNESCO now plays in the global struggle against HIV/AIDS.

Very special words of appreciation are due to Michael Morrissey who was an educational consultant in the UNESCO's Office for the Caribbean during the period of the book's genesis. His perceptive insights laid the foundation for the commencement of this work. His personal engagement ensured that the initial momentum was maintained. His unflagging encouragement nurtured the book's development through many difficult days. Without his interest and commitment the book would not have come into existence. The text may be ours, but the credit is his.

We wish to express our personal indebtedness to Hélène-Marie Gosselin, Director of the UNESCO's Office for the Caribbean, and Françoise Caillods, Deputy Director of the International Institute for Educational Planning (IIEP), for their unfailing encouragement and support. We thank Olatz Landa Pena, also from the UNESCO's Office for the Caribbean, who played a key role in facilitating our access to documentary sources. Gabriel Rugalema and Eric Allemano, both from the IIEP, provided insightful observations on the first draft of the manuscript. Inon Schenker, researcher, Hebrew University of Jerusalem, also read the manuscript and offered many pertinent suggestions. We are greatly indebted to these and to the many others who shared their time and expertise in meetings and discussions. Without their support the book could not have been written.

MAP OF THE CARIBBEAN

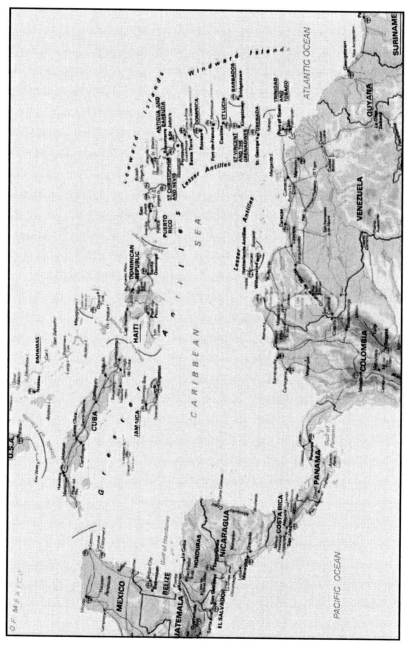

Source: Caribbean Junior Social Studies Atlas. London and Basingstoke: Macmillan Publishers, 1990.

INTRODUCTION

If, as has been said, the HIV/AIDS pandemic could well be Planet Earth's worst weapon of mass destruction endangering all of humankind, then the Caribbean in its new-found vulnerability needs to engage in a pre-emptive strike against ignorance, denial, stigma and discrimination which are themselves most effective agents contributing to the spread of AIDS.

George Alleyne, Director Emeritus of the Pan American Health Organization (PAHO) and a former Professor of Medicine in the University of the West Indies, cited the Director of UNAIDS who in addressing a joint session of Jamaica's parliament in 2002 said that the AIDS epidemic 'requires appropriate social policies and a legal framework so that organising against AIDS is supported, and the corrosive impact of discrimination countered, including [that] against those groups and individuals in society who are most vulnerable to AIDS. George Alleyne himself expressed his wish to see the region emancipate itself 'from the mental slavery that results in homophobia and discrimination against persons who are perceived as having a lifestyle of which we do not approve'. There is enough to justify this appeal against the stigma that the AIDS pandemic engenders throughout the region. This can be seen in the ingrained religion supported by Old Testament texts, in the budding tradition of Jamaican dance-hall culture among pop musicians calling for death to those deemed to have sinful sexual orientations, and in the entrenched patriarchy syndrome evident everywhere, albeit in a strongly matriarchal Caribbean society.

The fact that the disease is no longer gender-specific is of particular importance in the Caribbean today where the highest recorded number of HIV/AIDS cases is not among men who have sex with men (MSM) but among women of child-bearing age and heterosexual men. This is in itself a threat to the growth and development of an entire society doomed to witness large numbers of its new generation born dead or ready for their coffins since they would have become infected through the natural processes of child-bearing and breast-feeding.

At the Regional Meeting of Ministers of Education in Latin America and the Caribbean held in Havana in November 2002, there was ready recognition that education is integral to the fight against AIDS, and that the disease will not be overcome without the full involvement of the education sector. The Ministers present acknowledged that more could be done through the education of teachers and students to prevent the spread of HIV. They affirmed the need to provide support and care to affected educators and learners, and they recognized that creative measures are needed to reduce the impact of the epidemic on our education sectors.

This book, *Education and HIV/AIDS in the Caribbean* by Michael J. Kelly in collaboration with Brendan Bain, provides welcome guidelines for achieving these aims as the text addresses the three concerns highlighted in the Havana Accord, namely, the education of teachers and students to prevent the spread of HIV, the provision of support and care to affected educators and learners, and the need for creative measures to reduce the impact of the epidemic on our education sectors. Procrastination has already stolen too much of the time that is so vital to planning and action. We must therefore now forge ahead with a constructive, creative and realistic approach to HIV/AIDS education, starting with the very young, if we are to eradicate this modern day plague that is already threatening to decimate our best and brightest – the region's youth population.

Health and education, as I have often said, demand serious investment in the human resource since each has to do with the human being's trajectory of life from cradle to grave, from infancy to old age. Freedom from disease is closely related to freedom from ignorance and both lead to freedom from hunger. All three conditions – disease, ignorance and hunger – are the hallmarks of poverty, the alleviation and eradication of which have become 'big questions' on the global development agenda.

The development process only makes sense when human beings, in terms of their hopes and aspirations, or of ideas about self and perceptions of the world which they wish to tenant with dignity, are placed at the centre of the process. Good health, as a key index of the quality of life and as a positive measure of social capital, then takes on new life and meaning.

But education must not only be for the young. There is a need for greater *continuing* public education in health and healthcare. Affette McCaw-Binns, one of my colleagues in the University of the West Indies, observed that 'the control of the major chronic diseases will require *renewed* health promotion efforts at community level to bring about the lifestyle changes needed to reduce the risks associated with the development of HIV' (my emphasis).

Education at all ages is therefore needed to dispel the myths and allay the fears associated with HIV/AIDS. Already the myth that sexual intercourse with a virgin will cure sexually transmitted diseases (STDs), has led to the spread of infection amongst young girls and the devastating effects of rape have been extended to include HIV/AIDS. In Jamaica HIV infection amongst girls is higher than for boys in the age group 9 to 13 years. This cannot be accounted for by transfer from the mother. Throughout the region, from the Bahamas to Trinidad and Tobago, a large number of children are infected with the virus, contributing their own share to the 2 to 3 percentage indicator of the HIV prevalence rate among the region's population.

The medical history of humanity is the story of the struggles of science with the workings of nature. Twenty-five million people were killed in six months during the global flu epidemic in 1918. The power of disease to mask its own mysteries has been re-asserted in our own time by AIDS.

In the Caribbean the spread of the HIV virus leading to the dreaded disease of AIDS is second only to what is occurring in southern Africa, the epicentre of the malady. The social and economic implications are far reaching since the disease threatens to deprive the entire region of much of its youth population who are the heirs to the legacy of achievement over generations and of the meaningful development now demanded of those very youths. The HIV/AIDS pandemic is to this generation of Caribbean people what tuberculosis was to mine. It threatens not only the immune system but also, in development terms, the region's productivity and economic potential. The lifeline tourist industry, which in some places has been accused of being the chief conduit of the dreaded disease, readily comes to mind.

The Pan American Health Organization (PAHO) a few years ago sent a wake-up call to the English-speaking Caribbean whose youthful populations were and still are in clear danger of massive premature losses, with the spread of the disease among young men, young women of child-bearing age, and children born to mothers with the HIV virus. The region is in danger of replicating the tragedy of southern Africa by being robbed of its youth, with tens of thousands of children orphaned and left to bring themselves up as best they can. The estimated climb in the number of children orphaned by AIDS, from 0.2 per cent of all children in 1980 to 3.2 per cent in 2010 for 10 Caribbean countries (*Chapter 8*) augurs ill for a future society whose growth will depend on the wellness of a productive workforce.

This book provides the information and impetus to face the fundamental challenge of educating our people about themselves, about AIDS, and about delivering health-care to themselves.

This process is not new, but needs to be re-institutionalized and revitalized in the education system. Throughout rural and urban Caribbean, during the early post-World War II years and even before, children of my generation were taught fantastic lessons in preventive medicine, albeit in basic form. As we were so often told, 'prevention is better than cure'. Before drinking water, we boiled it whenever the river was in spate. Spitting in public, sharing eating utensils, not washing hands before eating or preparing food, allowing stagnant water to form mosquito breeding places, were all known to spread disease. At school, fingernails and hair were examined at morning assemblies. We learnt to clean our teeth with chew sticks as healthy teeth and gums aided in mastication and the digestion of food.

The eradication, or near eradication, of typhoid, yaws, malaria, and tuberculosis was the result of information that flooded the primary school classrooms about these communicable and chronic diseases and the remedies for prevention and cure. There is a need for such a programme of health science in our primary schools, to teach the basic tenets of personal hygiene, to alert the student population at a very early age to the increasing incidence of HIV infection, especially at a time when there is much pregnancy amongst school girls, and to affirm the presence of malnutrition and the threatened resurgence of diseases such as tuberculosis that were once held in check. This book is a timely tool for intervention through public education.

I am heartened that *Education and HIV/AIDS in the Caribbean* gives direction as to how to reach the thousands of persons who are not in the formal education system, and are themselves most vulnerable, for example, street children, the homeless and those incarcerated. It also tackles the devastating social consequences of AIDS that we in the region face and the special needs of orphans and children made vulnerable by the disease.

I congratulate Michael Kelly, a tireless worker and educator in Zambia and a man of enormous compassion, for this succinct text and Brendan Bain of the UWI who gave critical support. Taken seriously by our educators and health personnel, it provides a road map to prevention even if it is not yet a total cure. For the threat of annihilation is a shockingly awesome thing to contemplate let alone to witness. The very thought indeed tempts one to keep wondering whether the pandemic is not truly the worst and vilest weapon of mass destruction that the world has ever experienced, one that deserves more attention, untied financial assistance from the 'first world', and far more structured public education across the entire world than it now receives.

Rex Nettleford
Vice Chancellor, University of the West Indies

THE HIV/AIDS EPIDEMIC

CHAPTER 1

The Global HIV/AIDS Epidemic

Global resolve

In January 2000, the United Nations Security Council signalled international recognition of the security implications of HIV/AIDS by holding a debate on the epidemic. This was its first ever debate on a health or development issue, and the first of many high level AIDS related meetings, held at intervals throughout 2000 and 2001. Thus in July 2000, the heads of government of the Caribbean Community (CARICOM) publicly recognised that the epidemic threatened to reverse the development achievements that the region had achieved in the previous three decades, and followed this up with the establishment in February 2001 of the Pan-Caribbean Partnership Against HIV/AIDS (PANCAP).

In a somewhat similar vein, in the Abuja Declaration of April 2001 African heads of state recognised that the epidemics of HIV/AIDS, tuberculosis and other related infectious diseases, through their potential to undermine development, social cohesion, political stability, and food security, constituted not only a major health crisis, but also the greatest global threat to the survival and life expectancy of the peoples of Africa. The Abuja Declaration was significant in being accompanied by a framework for action and mechanisms for monitoring how the plan was being implemented.

Similar commitments and undertakings appeared in the Baltic States Declaration (May 2000), the Declaration of the Tenth Ibero-

American Summit of heads of state (November 2000), the regional call to fight HIV/AIDS in Asia and the Pacific (April 2001), the European Union Programme for Action (May 2001), and the Central Asian Declaration on HIV/AIDS (May 2001).

These regional expressions of concern culminated in June 2001 at the United Nations General Assembly Special Session (UNGASS) on HIV/AIDS when the world established a global alliance against the epidemic with a solemn commitment to address the HIV/ AIDS crisis with intensified action and increased resources. A practical outcome was progress in establishing the Global Fund to Fight AIDS, Tuberculosis and Malaria (GFATM), an innovative and independent, public-private partnership. The aims of GFATM are to increase global resources to combat the three diseases, direct these resources where they are needed most, and ensure that they are used effectively.

The global scale and scope of HIV/AIDS

The continued spread of HIV/AIDS has made such intensified political momentum vitally important. The new millennium saw evidence that Senegal, Thailand and Uganda were consolidating early successes in confronting the epidemic, and were being joined very gradually by countries such as Cambodia, South Africa and Zambia. It also saw Botswana and Brazil addressing the epidemic in comprehensive care and prevention programmes that showed success in reducing the number of AIDS deaths and new HIV infections.

Successes in responding to the epidemic are of immense significance in reducing suffering and setbacks for affected individuals and for the communities and countries concerned. They are also significant in demonstrating that success against HIV/AIDS is possible.

But the success stories are overshadowed by the relentless growth in the scale and scope of the epidemic. Almost every passing year sees a revision upwards of HIV/AIDS estimates and projections. The way the disease continues to outstrip even the most pessimistic projections reveals two features that are of consequence in every effort to get to grips with it. First, the opening years of the twenty-first century saw the world still experiencing what was clearly an early phase of the epidemic. Prevalence levels climbed higher than previously believed possible in the worst affected countries, while the disease continued to spread rapidly into new populations in Africa, Asia, the Caribbean and Eastern Europe, particularly in heavily populated countries. Second, HIV/AIDS is showing itself to be an ever changing epidemic, manifesting itself in different ways in different situations. Its outcomes are complex and surprising. It is not possible to anticipate all of them. Hence every response, including those made by the education sector, should be flexible enough to accommodate the unexpected.

The epidemic has spared no country in the world. In the majority, its prevalence is still at a low level. At the end of 2001, the adult prevalence rate[1] was below one per cent in two-thirds of the 147 countries for which data were available (UNAIDS, 2002a). But this gives no cause for complacency since experience with the epidemic in the first quarter century of its manifestation has shown the rapid violence with which it can explode. Moreover, low prevalence at national level can conceal pockets where the rate is high, as is the case in China where the national prevalence of 0.1 per cent does not adequately capture the extent of the disease in provinces such as Yunnan and Henan, and the serious localized epidemics occurring among certain population groups. In addition, even with low prevalence rates, the numbers infected may be very large, depending on the size of the population. Thus, at the end of 2001, it was estimated that there were 3,970,000 adults and children living with HIV/AIDS in India where the reported prevalence rate was 0.8 per cent, compared with 330,000 in Botswana, where the reported prevalence rate of 38.8 per cent was one of the highest in the world.

In 24 countries, however, the adult prevalence rate at the end of 2001 lay between 1 and 5 per cent and in a further 25 it was 5 per cent or higher. Apart from Haiti, countries with prevalence levels above 5 per cent were all in sub-Saharan Africa. Intermediate prevalence levels were also found in several African countries, as well as in the Caribbean (three countries), South East Asia (two countries), Eastern Europe (two countries), and Latin America (six countries).

In the majority of these countries, the extent of the AIDS epidemic is estimated by adjusting data originating in antenatal and sexually transmitted infection (STI) clinics (sentinel surveillance data). The limitations of this method have led some high prevalence countries to undertake actual HIV testing as an integral part of routine population surveys. These surveys tend to find prevalence rates that are lower than those estimated on the basis of the antenatal clinic data, though still alarmingly high (for instance, in Zambia, the survey data yielded a prevalence rate of 15.6 per cent, compared with a rate of 21.5 per cent on the basis of sentinel surveillance data. For South Africa the corresponding figures were 11.4 per cent from survey data and 20.1 per cent from sentinel surveillance data). Previous estimates may have exaggerated somewhat the scale of the epidemic, but the more realistic survey estimates do not give grounds for much comfort.

Global projections

The projections in relation to the development of the epidemic have both spatial and temporal dimensions. Spatially, or geographically, the epicentre of the epidemic could move from its current location in southern and eastern Africa to east or south Asia. Both India and China are reported to be on the brink of AIDS crises of titanic dimensions that would result in unimaginable suffering, economic loss and social devastation. Already, India is said to be on an HIV/AIDS trajectory similar to that found in Africa 15 years earlier. The Russian Federation is experiencing a rapidly developing epidemic (at the time of writing, the fastest growing in the world), with the number of infected persons projected to increase within 7 to 10 years to about twice the total number currently infected in South Africa. But although Africa might no longer be the epicentre of the epidemic, the projections for Nigeria and Ethiopia, two of its most populous countries, are bleak, with the possibility of already high prevalence rates doubling or even trebling and the number of infected persons increasing to more than seven million in each country. If the epidemic progresses along these lines in these countries, it will bring unprecedented human suffering, decimate key government and business elites, undermine growth and dismantle the prospects for human and economic development (Gordon, 2002).

The temporal aspect of HIV/AIDS is that in a very short space of time it has swept across the world, becoming in less than 25 years an epidemic of worldwide proportions. It arrived quickly and with dramatic speed began unravelling development gains that had been arduously won over several decades. But its departure will not be as quick. Experience shows that most prevention programmes are slow in stemming transmission of the virus. Projections are that an additional 45 million people will become infected with HIV between 2002 and 2010, unless the world succeeds in mounting a drastically expanded global prevention effort (UNAIDS, 2002b: 5). On the basis of experience to date, it seems unlikely that the epidemic will peak worldwide until the second half of the twenty-first century (Feachem, 2003). By then there could be a staggering 30 to 140 million persons living with HIV/AIDS in India alone and 32 to 100 million in China (Eberstadt, 2002). Even if these new waves of the epidemic could be rolled back (something that currently seems very unlikely) and the incidence of new HIV infections were to be dramatically reduced, a very large proportion of the 40 million individuals who are already infected will very likely die within a few years. This loss of millions of individuals in their most productive years will further constrain development efforts. It will also increase the number of orphans and aggravate the challenge they pose.

In this light, HIV/AIDS-affected countries that became politically independent in the middle of the twentieth century must face the hard reality that the day of their independence from HIV/ AIDS is likely to lie much further away in the future than when they gained political independence. They need to be prepared for a long-term commitment and for interventions that will extend across one generation or more.

This long-term perspective has immediate relevance for the education sector. As will be seen in subsequent chapters, the effective response of the sector to the epidemic necessitates innovative and comprehensive management, and curriculum and teacher preparation measures. The persistence of the epidemic and its impacts will energize policy-makers and planners to be resolute in ensuring that these measures are long-term, substantive and effective. Educational responses to the epidemic almost certainly will be required until well into the second half of this century.

One of the most salient features of the HIV disease is that it has no cure at present. Once established, in an individual or community, it remains permanent. Antiretroviral therapy can suppress the activity of the virus within the human body, extend an individual's life prospects, and make it possible for the infected person to live a fulfilling, productive, complete human life. This accommodation with the disease can be so life-enhancing that it should be available to every infected person. At the time of writing, intensive consideration is being given to issues relating to the production, pricing, affordability, distribution and use of antiretroviral drugs. The aim is to ensure that every person who needs it has access to this form of therapy. Progress in this direction will change the situation for the better, engender the conviction that the epidemic can be overcome, and strengthen the resolve to take the necessary action.

However, the therapy cannot eliminate the virus from within the body. The person never ceases to be infected. The virus remains latent as long as the infected person adheres to the required treatment regime, but quickly becomes active and virulent again when treatment is discontinued. The risk always remains that this resurgence of viral activity will recur. The infected person never succeeds in building up full protective immunity against a virus that, in turn, undermines the body's capacity to respond to other invasive organisms.

Faced with a galloping epidemic that has no cure and for which treatment is costly, unending, difficult to access and sometimes associated with harmful side effects, the world has sought to develop vaccines that would be safe, effective, and accessible, either in preventing HIV infection (preventive or prophylactic vaccines) or in suppressing HIV activity within the body (therapeutic vaccines). The thrust of research into the development of an HIV vaccine continues to gain momentum, with optimism that the eventual outcomes will be successful. Some researchers have expressed confidence that the fourth decade of HIV/AIDS, beginning about 2010, will see the availability of a vaccine that would provide complete protection against HIV. But success in vaccine development continues to elude science, with large-scale trials of candidate vaccines proving largely ineffective. To add to the problem, even if a vaccine were developed, the regulatory requirements imposed by different countries, pricing and production issues, and distribution constraints could result in long delays between the development of a vaccine and its extensive use in the world's most severely affected countries.

The many faces of HIV/AIDS

HIV/AIDS is an epidemic with many faces. Although referred to as if it were a single entity, in reality it consists of two bio-medical epidemics and two associated social epidemics occurring in sequence and eventually overlapping. First, there is the silent, invisible epidemic of HIV infection that, in most countries, is spread mainly by sexual activity. The deterioration of the human immune system in a person infected with HIV is long, slow and seldom detected. For several years the infected person may show no symptoms of being diseased. But all the while the virus remains active within the body. This viral activity leads to a progressive weakening and ultimate breakdown in the body's defence system. Throughout what may be a lengthy period of progressive deterioration, the virus can be transmitted through body fluids from the infected person to others. From the time of first infection, the infected person, though showing no symptoms, can be a source of HIV infection for others. This is a crucial feature that makes a salient contribution to the transmission of the disease.

The second part of the sequence is the highly visible epidemic of AIDS, the acquired immuno-deficiency syndrome. When the deterioration of the immune system reaches a certain degree, the person begins to experience, with increasing frequency, periodic bouts of illnesses and infections which an uninfected body would normally be able to ward off or cope with. Because of the impact of the HIV infection, the individual lacks a viable immune response to these further infections. Because these new or reactivated infections use the opportunity provided by the body's weakened defence system to establish themselves, they are referred to as opportunistic infections. An individual who experiences the level of immuno-deficiency at which these opportunistic infections occur is said to have AIDS, the acquired immuno-deficiency syndrome. As well as making the body susceptible to a variety of infections, the weakened immune system reduces to such an extent the system's potential to recover from these infections that in the great majority of cases the person becomes steadily weaker and eventually dies. Most will die within eight to ten years from the time when they became infected, and many will die even sooner. In the absence of treatment, the period between the manifestation of what is called AIDS and death seldom lasts longer than two years.

AIDS, or the acquired immunodeficiency syndrome, also increases the incidence of certain forms of cancer – for example, in areas of the world where human papilloma virus (HPV) infection is prevalent, the incidence of cancer of the cervix, caused by HPV, increases in persons with HIV infection. If not detected early and treated aggressively, this form of cancer progresses more rapidly in persons with HIV/AIDS than in other patients and causes additional suffering and premature death. Cancers that occur more frequently in persons with AIDS than in the general population also include some types of lymphomas and Kaposi's sarcoma.

The third element of the HIV/AIDS sequence is the adverse social reactions, stigma and discrimination that persons living with HIV or AIDS frequently experience. The belief is widespread that infected persons 'deserve' their fate because of their drug using habits or 'promiscuous' sexual behaviour. The disease is also associated with fear – not merely fear of its ready transmission and lethal outcome, but also fear that one's HIV/AIDS status might be discovered by a spouse or in the workplace. This stigma is a very real obstacle to both prevention and care. In many of the hardest-hit countries, government officials and ordinary citizens – including those most affected by the epidemic – often continue to look the other way because of the rejection, discrimination and shame attached to HIV/AIDS (UNAIDS, 1998*b*: 13).

Discrimination against people who live with HIV/AIDS extends further than the social and community spheres. There are well-authenticated cases of individuals being denied medical care because of their HIV status, of employment being terminated or promotion denied on the same grounds, and of children being excluded from school because of HIV/AIDS in their families (*Box 1*). It has also been noticed in Africa that the stigmatization and discrimination may be greater against women than against men.

Box 1. The stigma and discrimination experienced by an AIDS widow

In India, Manpreet, a trucker's widow in western Punjab, and three of her four daughters, tested HIV-positive after her husband died of suspected AIDS. The local school expelled her elder girls; her infant daughter died; and her father-in-law threw her out, forcing her to live with her three surviving children in her father's one-room house.

Source: CDC HIV/STD/TB *Prevention News Update*, 7 January 2003.

This situation breeds silence about the disease. There is no sincere acknowledgment of its presence. A wall of silence surrounds it, publicly and privately. Fear of hostile social consequences of the type experienced by Manpreet (*Box 1*) breeds reluctance to get it out into the open. It is referred to by innuendoes and half-suggestions. It is concealed as TB or malaria or meningitis or, in the Caribbean, as cancer or just as 'a sickness'. This silence reinforces the sense of shame and fear at both personal and institutional levels, and this in turn leads to even greater silence and isolation. It all becomes so great that families, communities, the media, the public sector may try to behave as if AIDS did not exist.

To some extent silence and denial are a basic and protective human response to situations that are excessively stressful – 'humankind cannot bear too much reality'.[2] But trying to cover up the existence of AIDS, as still commonly occurs in families and communities, and even in some countries, will never lead to mastery over the disease or its impacts. The atmosphere of denial, silence and stigma provides a dark and fertile breeding ground for the further spread of the virus, since individuals are afraid to seek the help, and possibly the treatment, they need.

This silence is as great in education as in other spheres. It is one of the tasks of an education system in today's world to try to break through this barrier of silence that surrounds HIV/AIDS. Likewise, it is one of the tasks of the present volume to bring out into the open what the epidemic can do to education systems across the Caribbean. It is only when there is a clear acknowledgement of the potential and actual catastrophic impacts that HIV/AIDS can have on their education systems that countries will be energized to plan for dealing with and surmounting those impacts.

The three epidemics of HIV, AIDS and stigma were first classified in this way in 1988 by Jonathan Mann, the charismatic head of the Global Programme against AIDS (the United Nations programme that preceded the establishment of UNAIDS). Since the late 1990s awareness has grown that a fourth AIDS-related epidemic stalks the world – the social epidemic of the vast number of children that the disease plunges into orphanhood, poverty and untold human misery. The number of orphans in the world today is almost unbelievably large. Not all are as a result of AIDS, but the proportion of children who have been orphaned by AIDS is increasing, while the proportion who have been orphaned by other causes is decreasing. It was estimated that by the end of 2001, there would be over 14 million children aged 15 or less in the world who had lost one or both parents to AIDS – a number that is projected to balloon to 25 million by 2010

(UNAIDS/UNICEF/USAID, 2002). The AIDS-generated orphans crisis bears so much on educational provision that it is dealt with separately in *Chapter 8* below.

The impact of HIV/AIDS on development

The world community has come to recognize that HIV/AIDS is not just a health problem. Much more, it is a development crisis of unprecedented proportions. In the face of the epidemic there is little hope that the epidemic development goals in the areas of human and economic well-being can be achieved. The disease reduces life expectancy; increases child mortality, leaves large numbers of children without adult care and places intolerable strains on health care systems. It undermines economic development through increased labour costs and the decreased availability of skilled human resources, and impoverishes households. Of special concern in the context of the interaction between the epidemic and education are its gender and poverty dimensions, variables that should not be viewed independently since in reality they interact in many ways.

AIDS and gender

The first cases of HIV/AIDS were detected in men, and during the first two decades of the epidemic more men than women were infected. But over time the proportion of infected women rose steadily in various parts of the world, with the result that the year 2002 saw global proportions of infected women and men being equal for the first time. The rapid increase in the proportion of infected women and girls means that they are experiencing an epidemic that is sweeping through them at a rate several times faster than that experienced by men and boys, a dynamic that seems set to continue. There are several reasons for this.

In the area of sexual relationships women enjoy less power than men and, for economic and emotional reasons, frequently experience coercion from their male partners. These factors increase their risk of becoming infected by an HIV-positive partner. Moreover, in heterosexual intercourse, transmission of HIV from male to female occurs more easily than that from female to male, partly because the surface area for contact with infected fluid is larger in the woman than in the man and partly because certain cells which are present in the lining of the female cervix (Langerhans' cells) provide a ready portal of entry for HIV. In addition to this, if a woman has intercourse with an HIV-infected person during her menstrual period, she is at increased risk of contracting the virus.

Patterns of sexual behaviour may add further to the infection risks experienced by women. In some parts of the world, including the Caribbean, there is evidence that some women have intercourse with bisexual males, some of whom are HIV-positive. Such men seldom disclose that they have multiple partners or that they are bisexual.

Because of a common pattern in which older men have sexual relations with younger women, and because of the relative vulnerability of women to HIV infection, young women are much more likely than young men to become infected. Data from virtually every country with prevalence above one per cent show that AIDS cases in young women aged 15 to 24 are more numerous than those in young men belonging to the same age group: At the end of 2001, the global picture was that for every 100 young men (aged 15 to 24) who were HIV-positive, there were 170 infected young women in the same age group (UNAIDS, 2002a). In several countries the situation was many times worse, with four to six times more young women than young men being infected.

This situation indicates that, as it progresses, HIV/AIDS is manifesting more of a feminine face. It is feasting on gender inequality and presaging catastrophe for families, communities and society. In many parts of the world, women are already cruelly disadvantaged by social, cultural and economic factors. The progress of the epidemic means that, in addition, many of them must carry the multiple burdens of HIV/AIDS. They experience it in their persons. They bear the responsibility of responding to its demands in their households and families. Even when ailing with the disease, they must attend to household chores, provide for their husbands and children, and engage in economic activity to ensure household needs.

Addressing gender inequalities is integral to addressing the HIV/ AIDS epidemic. But this also calls for a proper understanding of gender. There is a great need for theoretical and practical recognition that gender refers to men as well as to women. Hence programmes and interventions should keep two audiences in mind: women and girls on the one hand, in order to provide them with the social, economic and negotiating skills that will empower them to minimize their risk of HIV infection; men and boys on the other hand, so that a better understanding of their gender roles may lead to less dominance and more care and responsibility in their sexual behaviour.

To achieve this, education is necessary. Many of the important goals were spelled out at the World Education Forum held in Dakar in 2000:

- ensure that by 2015 all children, but especially girls, have access to and complete free primary education of good quality;

- achieve a 50 per cent improvement in levels of adult literacy by 2015, especially for women;

- eliminate gender disparities in primary and secondary education, and achieve gender equality in education by 2015, with a focus on ensuring girls' full and equal access to, and achievement in basic education of good quality.

Promoting universal access to good quality education and closing the gender gap at all levels of education are major steps in the right direction. But if education is to play a significant role in reducing the vulnerability of girls and young women to HIV infection, these steps need to be accompanied by sectorwide efforts to eliminate negative images and gender stereotypes, foster gender relevant knowledge, and promote appreciation of women's roles.

In contrast to many other parts of the world, closing the gender gap at all levels of education in the Caribbean involves ensuring the participation of boys and young men. This is an issue that the Caribbean as a region must address within the framework of the international Education For All (EFA) goal of the elimination of all gender-based disparities. But the region also experiences the need to move beyond the mere letter of the EFA goal, through policies and strategies that will encourage male teenagers and young men to remain in school to the end of the secondary cycle, to participate in tertiary-level programmes, and to undertake university studies.

AIDS and poverty

Unlike other infectious diseases, HIV/AIDS does not respect social barriers. It affects rich and poor alike. Nevertheless, poverty facilitates the transmission of HIV and its more rapid development into full-blown AIDS. One overarching reason for this is that in a situation of poverty, the urgency of responding to immediate short-term survival or satisfaction needs overrides concern about protecting conditions that lie several years in the future. This is very strongly the situation with HIV/AIDS, where no immediate harmful consequences are experienced and the infection appears to lie dormant for several years.

Poverty accentuates the vulnerability of the poor to HIV infection in a variety of interacting and accumulating ways. Those who are poor are more vulnerable to HIV infection because of:

- their lower nutritional status;
- their poorer state of general health, so that their immune system is already compromised;
- their increased exposure to other health hazards (malaria, tuberculosis, gastro-intestinal problems);
- their limited access to adequate health services;
- the smaller likelihood that they will seek or get treatment for sexually transmitted diseases with which they may be infected;
- their lack of access to information and the means of protecting themselves in sexual encounters;
- the greater likelihood that they will engage in risky sexual behaviour because of their limited ability to access condoms, store them properly, or use them correctly;
- the overcrowded conditions in which they live;

- the high risks to which they are exposed in providing care to HIV/AIDS patients in their homes;

- the survival needs which cause poor women and girls, as also poor men and boys, to enter into sexual relationships and to protect their expected income by not insisting on condom use;

- the economic needs which motivate young men from poor families to leave home and migrate to what may be high risk locales in search of work;

- the virtual absence of pleasurable experiences, other than sex, available to poor people.

At a deeper level, the vulnerability of the poor to HIV infection is heightened by their poverty. Compared with the more affluent, the poor have fewer choices, in relation to work, neighbours, housing, spending, or recreational activities. They experience uncertainty about their future and may not be conscious of the need to protect it. Pressures to meet immediate needs make potential AIDS impacts remote and unreal. Their living circumstances provide little opportunity for discussion with their partner about sex. In addition, the values, norms, codes and meanings by which the poor regulate their lives may never have assimilated HIV-prevention messages because these messages were communicated in a middle-class idiom that was alien to them. All of these circumstances combine to generate situations where the reality of HIV/AIDS may be acknowledged at the rational level, but ignored at the practical levels of living and behaving.

But if poverty exacerbates vulnerability to HIV/AIDS, the reverse is also true: HIV/AIDS aggravates poverty. It does so by thrusting households back on ever more limited resources as it removes wage-earners from employment, reduces the ability to engage in small-holding or agricultural work, deflects resources to medicines and health care, and draws down on savings or capital. The disease also aggravates the poverty situation through the reduction of employment opportunities as industry adjusts to its impact, while economic growth declines through the loss of skilled human resources and the use of resources for consumption rather than investment.

The vulnerability of the poor to HIV infection is accentuated for women and girls. Precisely because they are women, they are treated as if economically subordinate. Their access to capital and credit is limited. They carry most of the responsibility for ensuring that children are fed, educated and maintained in basic good health. In numerous cases, because of inadequate financial support from their partner, they have to apply their ingenuity and resources to maintaining their household, even to the extent of relying on the sale of sex to meet household survival needs. Pressures to meet their own immediate needs and those of their children far outweigh concerns that they might become HIV infected. Because they are poor women, they experience in themselves a double disadvantage, the feminisation of poverty and the feminisation of HIV/AIDS. This twofold disadvantage marks the urgency of ensuring that the potential of education is used to the full in dismantling the vicious cycle of poverty, gender inequality and HIV/AIDS (*Figure 1*). Above all, there is a need to ensure that every girl has access to quality education that will help her to emerge from the poverty trap, while equipping her with the values, attitudes, knowledge, and skills she needs to protect herself against HIV infection.

Figure 1. The central role of education in dismantling the vicious cycle of poverty, gender inequality, and HIV/AIDS

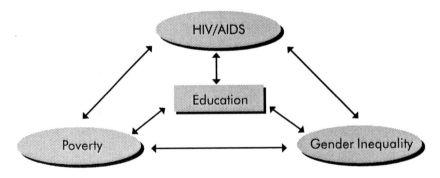

HIV/AIDS and human rights

HIV/AIDS makes an aggressive attack on the most basic of all human rights – the right to life that is enshrined in Article 3 of the Universal Declaration of Human Rights. But it makes equally aggressive attacks on a number of the other fundamental rights that the human family has endorsed:

- *The right to non-discrimination*: All human beings are born free and equal in dignity and rights (Article 1).

- *The right to education*: Everyone has the right to education (Article 26).

- *The right to information*: Everyone has the right to freedom of opinion and expression; this right includes freedom to hold opinions without interference and to seek, receive and impart information and ideas through any media and regardless of frontiers (Article 19).

- *The right to equality between men and women*: (a) Everyone is entitled to all the rights and freedoms set forth in this Declaration, without distinction of any kind, such as race, colour, sex, language, religion, political or other opinion, national or social origin, property, birth or other status (Article 2). (b) Men and women are entitled to equal rights as to marriage, during marriage and at its dissolution (Article 16).

- *The right to health*: Everyone has the right to a standard of living adequate for the health and well-being of himself and his family (Article 25).

- *The right to privacy*: No one shall be subjected to arbitrary interference with his privacy, family, home or correspondence, nor to attacks upon his honour and reputation (Article 12).

Significantly, in the late 1990s, UNAIDS and the Office of the United Nations High Commissioner for Human Rights issued joint international guidelines on HIV/AIDS and human rights and updated these four years later. In 1998, the two agencies jointly declared that 'an environment in which human rights are respected ensures that vulnerability to HIV/ AIDS is reduced, those infected with and affected by HIV/AIDS live a life of dignity without discrimination, and the personal and societal impact of HIV infection is alleviated' (UN, 1998: 5). In 2002 they went further by stating that 'human rights promotion and protection are central to the response to HIV/AIDS. Denying the rights of people living with HIV, and those affected by the epidemic, imperils not only their well-being, but life itself' (UN, 2002: 5).

A strong human rights approach to HIV prevention and to care and support for those who are infected or affected should lead to action along two dimensions:

1. The promotion of all that supports basic human rights, particularly the right to life, health, education, and gender equality.

2. The elimination of all forms and expressions of unfair discrimination.

One of the recurring themes of this book is the role that education must play in both of these areas. Education promotes understanding and practice in living together and experiencing shared purposes (UNESCO, 1996: 91-92). It develops in learners an appreciation of diversity and interdependence that respect the human worth of every person. It affirms in the strongest possible manner the inherent dignity of all human beings, no matter how diverse their qualities and characteristics, and emphasizes the need to support them in the untrammelled exercise of their human rights. In the area of HIV/ AIDS, it makes no room for stigma or discrimination, but through its teaching and practice seeks to communicate the simple but powerful message: 'my colleague with HIV/AIDS is still my colleague'.

Information, education and communication approaches to HIV/AIDS control

In contrast to bio-medical solutions that focus on a permanent cure, a vaccine, or adequate access to antiretroviral therapy, the standard approach to HIV/AIDS control has been to promote behaviour change and the adoption of skills that will reduce the likelihood of HIV infection, increase the prospect of more care and support, and seek to mitigate or manage the adverse impacts of the epidemic. This approach bases itself on information, education and communication (IEC) programmes that seek to bring about the desired individual, social and institutional changes. Many such programmes have been adopted in the education sector. However, the changes that they seek to produce are hard to achieve and slow to take effect.

IEC programmes need to be rooted in understandings that take adequate account of the context and socio-cultural milieu. Unfortunately, in the first two decades of the AIDS epidemic, the majority of these programmes tended to be based on theories, models and frameworks that derived principally from western perspectives and that were foreign to many non-western cultures. UNAIDS, the joint United Nations programme on HIV/AIDS, has found that the prevailing theories, models and assumptions tended to:

- focus on the individual rather than the social context;

- assume that HIV preventive decisions are based on rational volitional thinking – what George Bernard Shaw characterized as 'brute sanity'– to the exclusion of more true-to-life emotional responses, and that highly rational decision-making precedes sexual activity and risk-taking behaviour;

- cater for narrowly focused, short-term interests to the neglect of long-term, internally derived, broad-based solutions;

- assume that creating awareness will necessarily lead to behaviour change;

- focus very strongly on condom promotion without adequate attention to important aspects of the social context (UNAIDS, 1999b: 24-26).

Because they were based on assumptions and understandings that did not match the realities of the audiences to whom they were addressed, the IEC programmes of the 1980s and 1990s did not evolve from the meanings and values of the affected populations.

Consequently they had only limited success in addressing issues of prevention, stigma and discrimination, care and support, and impact mitigation. As a result of experience with earlier programmes, UNAIDS now advocates that communication strategies for HIV/AIDS prevention, care and support should focus attention on five interrelated contextual domains:

- Government policy – the role of policy and law in supporting or hindering prevention, care and support efforts.
- Socioeconomic status where account is taken of collective or individual income that may allow or prevent adequate intervention.
- Culture – the unique positive or negative characteristics that may promote or hinder prevention and care practices.
- Gender relations – the status of women in relation to men in society and community and the influence of this on sexual negotiation and decision-making.
- Spirituality – the role of spiritual and religious values in promoting or hindering the translation of prevention and care messages into positive actions (UNAIDS, 1999*b*: 29 ff).

For the foreseeable future, accelerating the disappearance of HIV/AIDS from the world will depend heavily on the adoption of the correct information, education and communication strategies. These are more likely to be successful in surmounting the multiple problems associated with HIV/AIDS if they are based in a communications framework that takes due account of the broad contextual domain in the way that UNAIDS has proposed. Hence the emphasis is shifting to IEC for social change, which empowers communities to deal with the issues of discrimination, poverty and gender inequality that drive the epidemic. As will appear in later chapters, this changing emphasis is as relevant for formal and non-formal educational programmes as it is for wider prevention and communication strategies.

The AIDS generation

Young people, living in the world of the twenty-first century, are the 'AIDS generation' (Kiragu, 2001: 1). They have never known a world without AIDS. For those in severely affected countries, AIDS is a fact of life, something that they see as having been there from the beginning and that many of them see as always being there. Their daily experience of sickness, death and funerals has numbed them into a terrible familiarity with suffering and an acceptance that this is the way things are. Their very immersion in the daily experience of the disease and its impacts and of the insufficient attempts to ensure prevention, treatment or care has made many of them distrustful of programmes and interventions. They feel overwhelmed by a constant barrage of prevention messages, many of them cast in forms which do not resonate. Many are suffering from 'AIDS fatigue', and turn away psychologically from efforts to reach them with new information, advice or products. Many are frankly cynical about the conflict they perceive between the messages being communicated to them and the behaviours and standards adopted by adults or portrayed in the media. Where circumstances allow the provision of antiretroviral therapy to the infected, the young are quick to spot the complacency that may subsequently develop – the idea that being HIV infected is not such a tragedy since it can be controlled by medication – and to internalize similar inappropriate attitudes. Recognition of these features is of importance in education.

At the beginning of 2002, about one-third of those living with HIV/AIDS were aged 15-24, while about half of all new adult infections were occurring among young people in this age range. In some countries it is projected that more than a third of the 15 year-olds will die of AIDS-related illnesses in the coming years. For countries with high rates of infection the prognosis is even worse. Thus, Zimbabwe may see half the 15-year old boys born in 1997 dying of AIDS before they reach the age of 50 (UNAIDS, 2000b: 25-26), while in the absence of treatment 90 per cent of Botswana girls and 88 per cent of the boys who were aged 15 in the year 2000 are likely to die of the disease (Kiragu, 2001). These young people, so many of whom seem almost inexorably destined for a premature death, are also the ones that the education sector seeks to reach, create a degree of consciousness, and assist.

The vulnerability of young people to HIV infection

Several physical, psychological and emotional factors make young people especially vulnerable to becoming infected with HIV. The lining of the genital tract of a girl is relatively immature and more delicate than that of an older woman, and the younger the girl, the smaller the genital aperture. Consequently, younger women are at greater risk than older women of trauma and bruising during sexual intercourse, factors that increase the likelihood of transfer of HIV from an infected male sexual partner. Coercion of young women by men, already alluded to as a frequent occurrence, increases these risks.

In addition to the direct physical risk for girls, both boys and girls lack experience and assurance in sexual relationships and, under pressure from their peers and the media, may feel an almost compulsive urge to experiment sexually without calculating the risk of contracting sexually transmitted infections. Yet another factor has to do with the poor nurturing of some young people, who have had little affirmation of their worth by their parents and other adults and who succumb to sexual advances by older individuals in an attempt to find affection and bolster their self-esteem.

A further characteristic feature of youth is a sense of invulnerability, the 'it won't happen to me' syndrome (and its fatalistic macho variation, the 'it doesn't matter if it happens to me' syndrome). Young people apply these attitudes to sexual encounters as readily as they do to fast driving or turning to alcohol or drugs for stimulation. At the beginning of 2002, Haiti's HIV prevalence rate of 6.1 per cent was the highest in the world outside of Africa. Yet in Haiti 63 per cent of sexually active girls aged 15-19 reportedly believe that they are not at risk of contracting the disease (UNICEF, 2000: 7).

Even though most young people allege that they know something about AIDS, many show themselves ignorant in ways that could be lethal for them. For instance, in several countries, including those with high prevalence rates, a significant proportion of youth report that they do not know any way of protecting themselves against infection. This was found to be the case for 51 per cent of girls and 35 per cent of boys aged 15-19 in Tanzania; in Bolivia, the percentages were 33 per cent for girls and 26 per cent for boys, while in Bangladesh the figures stood at the extraordinarily high level of 96 per cent for girls and 88 per cent for boys (UNICEF, 2000: 6). Another aspect of this potentially fatal lack of knowledge is the large number of young people who believe that HIV infection will show in the appearances of infected persons. Up to recently, in Viet Nam, 50 per cent of girls aged 15-19 said that they did not know that a person with HIV may look healthy. In Nepal, 80 per cent of girls of this age were reportedly unaware that a person who looks healthy can be infected with HIV and can transmit it to others (UNICEF, 2000: 7).

This ignorance extends to various areas of sexual activity. In Caribbean countries, where sexual activity begins at a young age, many young people seem to be well informed on HIV transmission, with almost all of them knowing that the virus is spread through sexual intercourse. According to their understanding, however, intercourse refers exclusively to vaginal penetration. They seem less aware that oral and anal intercourse and any other way of sharing bodily fluids also constitute high-risk activity.

A final area where the knowledge and sexual practices of youth may lead to disaster arises from the trust they show in each other and in older persons when they enter into a relationship: establishing a special intimate relationship is a wonderful and very beautiful thing, something that is so valuable and marvellous that it needs to be safeguarded. Many counsellors recommend that young people should strive to build friendship and trust over time before moving to the stage of sexual intercourse. When physical intimacy precedes trust, risk is higher, and the likelihood of transmitting infections from previous or concurrent partnerships is greater. Ideally, and especially in the age of HIV/AIDS, commitment to mutual fidelity should precede sexual intercourse. Where intercourse comes first, then the use of a condom or other barrier method is strongly advised to greatly reduce the risk of HIV transmission. Frequently, however, young people are reluctant to wait. They are often also reluctant to use condoms partly because they feel that this would indicate a lack of trust in their partner. And in several instances, they may stop using condoms after some weeks or months of a relationship, protesting that there is no longer any need, that they are faithful to each other. What they often do not know is whether that fidelity is absolute, and also what the sexual history of the partner was before they came together.

These illustrations and situations show that ignorance about HIV risks is very widespread, especially in the early years of sexual activity. Notwithstanding the 'AIDS fatigue' experienced by many, much more needs to be done to ensure that young people are provided with accurate information and to keep them alert to the risks they might encounter. As UNICEF rightly says, 'the overwhelming message is that information about AIDS and its deadly danger is not getting out or is not being absorbed' (UNICEF, 2000: 6). A major thesis of this book is that the education sector has a responsibility to ensure that correct information reaches young people around the world in ways that will speak to them, and that will help them make these messages their own.

Notes

1. The adult prevalence rate is the estimated number of persons aged 15 to 49 years who are living with HIV or AIDS divided by the mid-year population of persons aged 15 to 49 years, for the year in question.
2. T. S. Eliot, *Four Quartets*.

CHAPTER 2

The HIV/AIDS Epidemic in the Caribbean

The Caribbean context

The Caribbean is a very heterogeneous region comprising some 30 territories with about 36 million inhabitants (*Box 2*). Territories vary widely in size and population, with Cuba being the largest (110,860 square kilometres, population 11,260,000) and Anguilla the smallest (96 square kilometres, population 8,000). As with Cuba, the populations of the Dominican Republic, Haiti, Puerto Rico, Jamaica, and Trinidad and Tobago all exceed one million, whereas the populations of the other territories are less than one million (*Table 1*). With a combined population of almost 28 million, three countries – Cuba, the Dominican Republic, and Haiti – between them account for about three-quarters of the entire population of the Caribbean.

Cuba, the Dominican Republic and Puerto Rico are Spanish-speaking; French is the official language of Haiti, French Guyana, and the French overseas territories of St. Martin, Guadeloupe, and Martinique; and Dutch is the official language in Suriname, Aruba, and the Netherlands Antillean Island Territories. All other territories are English-speaking. With the exception of those that are United States territories, the English-speaking countries are all members of the Commonwealth and are sometimes referred to as the Commonwealth Caribbean.

Table 1. Countries and territories of the Caribbean

Country or territory	Area (square kilometres)	Population	Net primary school enrolment rate (%)	Adult literacy rate (%)	Life at expectancy birth (years)	GNI per capita (US dollars)
Anguilla	96	8,000	N/A	95.0	77	N/A
Antigua & Barbuda	442	68,000	N/A	89.0	75	9,150
Aruba	193	96,000	97.0	97.0	79	N/A
The Bahamas	13939	309,000	83.0	95.4	69	12,270
Barbados	430	280,000	89.7	99.7	76	9,280
Belize	22.965	250,000	100.0	93.2	74	3,110
British Virgin Islands	153	22,000	N/A	98.0	76	N/A
Cayman Islands	259	38,000	N/A	98.0	80	N/A
Cuba	110,860	11,260,000	99.2	96.7	N/A	N/A
Dominica	750	72,000	N/A	94.0	74	N/A
Dominican Republic	48.442	8,700,000	90.6	83.7	67	2,130
Grenada	345	95,000	81.0	98.0	73	3,720
Guadeloupe	1,780	455,000	N/A	90.0	78	N/A
Guyana	214,969	725,000	N/A	98.5	63	860
Haiti	27,750	8,000,000	N/A	49.8	54	510

Jamaica	10,991	2,750,000	94.2	86.9	75	2440
Martinique	1,128	420,000	N/A	93.0	79	N/A
Montserrat	102	4,000	N/A	97.0	79	N/A
Netherlands Antillean Island Territories	800	205,000	95.0	96.5	76	N/A
Puerto Rico	8,959	3,960,000	N/A	89.0	76	N/A
St. Kitts & Nevis	262	41,000	N/A	97.0	71	6,880
St. Lucia	616	150,000	95.7	67.0	71	3,970
St. Martin	54	35,000	N/A	N/A	N/A	N/A
St. Vincent and the Grenadines	389	115,000	N/A	96.0	73	2,690
Suriname	163,300	400,000	98.0	93.0	70	1,660
Trinidad & Tobago	5,128	1,330,000	92.9	98.3	73	4930
Turks & Caicos	430	15,000	N/A	98.0	74	N/A
Virgin Islands of the United States	347	110,000	N/A	98.0	78	N/A

Sources: Longman, *Caribbean School Atlas*, Third Edition; World Bank Country Fact Sheets; *Global EFA Monitoring Report 2002.*

Box 2. The Caribbean.

Definitions of the territorial scope of the Caribbean vary. Probably the 'socio-cultural' definition of the 'wider' Caribbean is most relevant as it pertains to the HIV/AIDS epidemic within the region. The 'wider' Caribbean region includes the following:

1. Fourteen sovereign state members of the Caribbean Community (CARICOM), including both island nations (Antigua and Barbuda, The Bahamas, Barbados, Dominica, Grenada, Haiti, Jamaica, Saint Kitts and Nevis, Saint Lucia, Saint Vincent and the Grenadines, and Trinidad and Tobago) and the mainland countries of Belize in Central America, and Guyana and Suriname in South America.

2. Spanish-speaking Cuba and the Dominican Republic.

3. Two semi-autonomous states of the Kingdom of the Netherlands (Aruba and the Netherlands Antillean Island Territries of Bonaire, Curacao, St. Martin, Statia, and Saba).

4. Six British Overseas Territories of Anguilla, Bermuda*, British Virgin Islands, Cayman Islands, Montserrat**, and the Turks and Caicos Islands.

5. The U.S. Commonwealth of Puerto Rico and territory of the U.S. Virgin Islands.

6. Four territories of the Republic of France consisting of French Guyana*, St. Martin, Guadeloupe, and Martinique.

*   Bermuda and French Guyana are not usually classified as part of the Caribbean.

**   Montserrat is also a member of CARICOM.

Source: Based on Table 2-1 of *HIV/AIDS in the Caribbean: Issues and Options.* Human Development Sector Management Unit, World Bank, June 2000.

Though formally classified as 'developing', the majority of Caribbean countries show quite high levels of human development in terms of life expectancy, school enrolment rates and adult literacy, three of the four indicators that combine to form the human development index (HDI; *Table 2*).[1] In 1999, Barbados and Bahamas ranked among the 48 countries in the world with the highest levels of human development (HDI > 0.800); Haiti, ranking 134 out of the 162 countries for which the HDI was available, was the only country in the region to be classified among the 36 countries with low human development levels (HDI < 0.500), while the remainder of the Caribbean countries for which information was available ranked among the 78 with medium human development levels. If full data were available for life expectancy, education enrolment rates, adult literacy levels, and per capita GDP in the island states for which HDI data are not published, they would probably all rank with countries at medium levels of human development, while the relatively high per capita GDP of some might place them with Barbados and Bahamas among the countries with the highest levels of human development in the world.

Table 2. Human Development Index for selected Caribbean countries, 1999

	Human Development Index (HDI)	HDI rank (among 162 countries)
The Bahamas	0.820	42
Barbados	0.864	31
Belize	0.776	54
Dominican Republic	0.722	86
Guyana	0.704	93
Haiti	0.467	134
Jamaica	0.738	78
Suriname	0.758	64
Trinidad & Tobago	0.798	49

Source: UNDP, *Human Development Report 2001*: 141-144.

At the beginning of the twenty-first century, per capita Gross National Income ranged from US$510 in Haiti to US$12,270 in Bahamas, the median for the 14 countries for which data is available being US$3,415 (*Table 1*). Throughout the 1990s the region's average economic growth rate was about two per cent. Economic activity in the region varies and includes the export of petroleum from Trinidad and Tobago, bauxite from Suriname, Guyana and Jamaica, and bananas from the small island territories of the Organization of Eastern Caribbean States (OECS).[2] The region receives more than 20 million visitors from abroad each year, making it one of the most popular tourist destinations in the world. Tourism is of special importance in OECS territories where it accounts for more than half the value of the GDP.

An important feature of the region (and one that has special relevance for HIV transmission) is the mobility of people. Notwithstanding the costs and logistics involved, there is considerable movement of people from island to island and outside the region for work, study and family reasons. People may also move across land borders, as between Haiti and the Dominican Republic, or Guyana and Suriname, even though this entails adapting to a different language. As a result of migration out of the region, significant numbers from the Caribbean have migrated to the United Kingdom, Holland, France and North America and there are smaller scatterings of people of Caribbean origin in many other parts of the world. Especially where large numbers of migrants have settled, people from the Caribbean tend to retain their Caribbean cultural identity. This Caribbean diaspora is important as a source of financial remittances to relatives who have not migrated out of their country of origin and in facilitating the movement of family members in and out of the region. In addition, members of the diaspora often invest in business entities and influence political decision-making in their home countries.

Religion and music are significant factors throughout the region. Religious organisations have played a prominent part in the development of the school systems in nearly every Caribbean country.

Faith-based organisations have also contributed greatly to the establishment of hospitals, and more recently in some countries they have been helping to supplement the delivery of primary health care through the establishment of low-cost drop-in clinics. In addition, religious authorities are widely respected and the views of their spokespersons are considered with care.

Because the majority of Caribbean people have common ancestral origins, there are similarities in many of their cultural expressions, such as music, dance and art. In many respects, music and dance are the lingua franca of the region. The vitality and creativity of the musical and artistic forms that have been created by Caribbean artistes are witness to the vitality and creativity that characterize the peoples of the region. A tangible manifestation of this creativity is the Caribbean introduction to the world of the steel band, the only new musical form created during the twentieth century.

The HIV/AIDS epidemic

The Caribbean is seriously affected by HIV/AIDS, with an overall prevalence rate of 2.3 per cent at the end of 2001, an estimated 429,000 adults (and 20,000 children) throughout the region living with the disease, and AIDS being the leading cause of death in the 15 to 44 age group (*Table 3*). No country has been spared. By the end of 1985, every Caribbean country had reported at least one AIDS case. AIDS incidence rates (the number of new cases occurring in a specified period of time) show a strong upward trend in all countries, with more cases being reported in the region between 1995 and 1998 than the cumulative total for all of the preceding years since the first manifestation of the epidemic in the early 1980s.

Table 3. HIV data for selected Caribbean countries (at the end of 2001)

Country	Adult (15-49) HIV prevalence rate (%)	Total number of adults infected (15-49 years)	Female infections (% of adults infections)	AIDS orphans (number of currently living children aged 0-14 who have lost one or both parents to AIDS)
The Bahamas	3.5	6,100	44.3	2,900
Barbados	1.2	2,000	No data	No data
Belize	2.0	2,200	45.5	950
Cuba	<0.1	3,200	25.9	1,000
Dominica	2.5	120,000	50.8	33,000
Guyana	2.7	17,000	50.0	4,200
Haiti	6.1	240,000	50.0	280,000
Jamaica	1.2	18,000	40.0	5,100
Suriname	1.2	3,600	50.0	1,700
Trinidad and Tobago	2.5	17,000	32.9	3,600
Caribbean countries	2.3	429,100	48.8	332,450

Source: UNAIDS, Epidemiological Fact Sheets, 2002 Updates, for each country

The information given in *Table 3* reveals a wide variation in prevalence within the region, ranging from a high of 6.1 per cent in Haiti to less than 0.1 per cent in Cuba. Nevertheless, there is no clear picture on just how extensive the disease is across the wider Caribbean. The fact that information can be given for only ten countries points to a major data limitation. Surmounting this limitation is not easy for the small island states that still need to increase their numbers of trained staff and deploy more resources in order to ensure comprehensive and reliable data collection. A further limitation is that most of the data on HIV/AIDS in the Caribbean is based on reporting of AIDS cases, and not on HIV status. Because AIDS-related stigma and discrimination are rampant throughout the region, there is considerable under-reporting of such cases. In addition, many AIDS diagnoses and much treatment take place in private facilities or outside the country to which the person belongs, and hence are not included in official statistics.

It is generally acknowledged that these limitations and weak HIV surveillance systems make it difficult to gauge the actual size of the HIV/AIDS problem in the Caribbean and it may be larger than the published statistics indicate. Adjusting official statistics for underreporting, UNAIDS estimated in 2000 that the officially reported figures should be adjusted upwards by about 40 per cent. Applying this adjustment to the number of reported cases at the end of 2001 would mean that there were about 600,000 adults in the Caribbean infected with HIV/AIDS, giving an adult infection rate of 3.2 per cent. Very likely, the rate would be found to be even higher if estimates were based on more systematic and up-to-date sentinel surveillance reports.

It is frequently stated that, after Sub-Saharan Africa where the adult HIV prevalence rate is 9.0 per cent, no region in the world is affected by HIV/AIDS as severely as the Caribbean. This is true, but perhaps just as telling are comparisons at the global level. At the end of 2001, the global HIV infection rate for adults aged 15 to 49 was 1.2 per cent; in the Caribbean it was almost two times larger at 2.3 per cent, and if the adjustments for under-reporting were taken into account it would have been almost three times larger at 3.2 per cent. The Caribbean is two to three times more severely HIV/AIDS infected than the world at large.

The relatively low-prevalence[3] setting that characterises some Caribbean countries does not justify complacency. UNAIDS has pointed out that 'all countries have, at some point in their epidemic histories, been low-prevalence countries' (UNAIDS, 2001: 5). The dramatic speed with which a low prevalence situation can change is demonstrated by South Africa. HIV prevalence among women attending antenatal clinics in South Africa was less than one per cent in 1990. Ten years later it was more than 24 per cent. The course of the epidemic in other countries could be similar, with a rapid escalation of prevalence where steps are not taken to contain the disease.

The epidemic has become firmly rooted in the general population in The Bahamas, Barbados, Belize, the Dominican Republic, Guyana, Haiti, Jamaica, Suriname, and Trinidad and Tobago. Official prevalence levels in all of these countries exceed one per cent of those between the ages of 15 and 49 (*Table 3*). In other words, there is a real likelihood that heterosexual spread of the epidemic is occurring in more than one per cent of the general population.

In the absence of the necessary testing and analysis, it is not possible to say whether the epidemic in the other Caribbean countries is generalized, concentrated, or nascent (the epidemic is said to be nascent when prevalence is less than five per cent in all known subpopulations presumed to practise high-risk behaviour). Limited information is available, however, for the 1996 HIV/AIDS incidence rate per 100,000 of the population for some of the countries in the Eastern Caribbean. For Antigua and Barbuda the rate was 204.9, for Dominica 207.6, for Grenada 189.6, for Montserrat 78.7, for St. Kitts and Nevis 145.0, for St. Lucia 94.0, and for St. Vincent and the Grenadines 160.6 (Theodore, 2000). Comparing these figures with similar data for countries where the HIV prevalence rate is known, the situation in all of these countries, with the exception of Montserrat and St. Lucia, would seem to be similar to that in Belize or Jamaica.

The picture from Cuba is strikingly different. At the end of 2001, just 0.03 per cent of the population of 11.26 million were HIV-positive. A wide-ranging prevention and treatment programme, backed by strong political action, has given Cuba the lowest levels of AIDS prevalence and HIV infection in the western hemisphere – and one of the lowest HIV-positive rates in the world. By comparison, the infection rate in the United States is fourteen times higher. Cuba's ability to contain the epidemic merits further investigation and the emulation of its success.

In the Caribbean, HIV is transmitted mainly through sexual practices. Heterosexual sexual activity is the dominant mode of transmission, accounting for about 60 per cent of the identified cases. Transmission by men who have sex with men is also considerable, accounting for at least a further 10 per cent (and approximately 20 per cent in the English-speaking Caribbean). Vertical transmission, from parent to child (PTCT), represents approximately six per cent of all reported AIDS cases and is the highest rate of PTCT in the western hemisphere. In more than one-fifth of the reported AIDS cases, the mode of HIV transmission is not known. Emerging evidence, in the Caribbean and elsewhere, on the extent of male bisexual practices, exposes a major transmission route for HIV infection from men who have sex with men to the general population.

Figure 2. Age of sexual initiation among 10-18 year-old school students in nine Caribbean countries

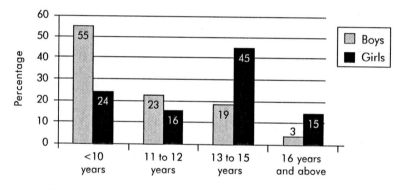

Source: *PAHO Adolescent Health Survey 2000* (Allen, 2002).

UNAIDS has noted that 'the heterosexual epidemics of HIV infection in the Caribbean are driven by the deadly combination of early sexual activity and frequent partner exchange by young people' (UNAIDS, 2000b: 18), and goes on to cite evidence from St. Vincent and the Grenadines showing that half of both men and women were sexually active at the age of 16. The mixing of ages – older men having sex with younger women – is common in many parts of the region and contributes to HIV rates being higher among young women than among young men belonging to the same age group.

Further evidence of early sexual activity comes from a cross-national study conducted among more than 15,000 school students aged 10 to 18 in nine English-speaking Caribbean countries. The investigation found that 55 per cent of boys and 24 per cent of girls reported having had sexual intercourse before the age of 10, while a further 23 per cent of boys and 16 per cent of girls indicated that they had initiated sexual activity between the ages of 11 and 12 (*Figure 2*). On the basis of these findings, 78 per cent of Caribbean boys and 40 per cent of girls become sexually active before they enter their teens.

Much of the Caribbean borders on major drug producing areas, and the region is of considerable importance in the transhipment of cocaine to Europe and North America. Surprisingly, therefore, the transmission of HIV by injecting drug use is reported to be small, accounting for no more than two per cent of AIDS cases. In support of this, medical practitioners confirm that, except in Puerto Rico, they see very few persons with marks on their bodies from the use of intravenous drugs. Also Caribbean people often acknowledge fear of needles and needle-sticks.

The feminine face of HIV/AIDS is becoming more visible in the Caribbean. In the early part of the 1990s, almost twice as many men as women were infected, but that picture has changed rapidly, resulting at the end of 2001 in 48.8 per cent of those living with HIV/AIDS in the region being women (*Table 3* above). As this can only come about if more women than men become infected, the change points to the assault that the epidemic is making on girls and young women. The especially vulnerable position of young women in the Caribbean is revealed by the estimates on HIV infection in young people aged 15 to 24: among young women in the region, the prevalence rate is estimated to lie in the range 1.8 to 3.2 per cent, whereas among young men in the same age group it is much lower, being estimated to lie between 1.4 and 2.4 per cent (UNAIDS, 2002*a*).

This development mirrors what is occurring elsewhere, with 2002 being a watershed year that saw parity in the number of HIV/AIDS cases between men and women worldwide. From this point forward, in the Caribbean and throughout the rest of the world, more women than men will be infected. Consider the cumulative adverse consequences this will have for mother-to-child transmission, family welfare, household production, and the enhancement of the dignity of women.

The impact of HIV/AIDS on Caribbean societies

Given that the picture of the extent of HIV/AIDS in the Caribbean is still relatively vague, it cannot be expected that the picture on the impact of the disease throughout the region will be any clearer. In addition, the long period that passes before HIV progresses to AIDS means that some of the social and economic consequences may not be felt immediately. However, because of the strong likelihood that the majority of persons who have contracted HIV infection will eventually die, it has been acknowledged that 'in the Caribbean, HIV/AIDS is a 'hurricane disaster' ... In fact, it is worse than hurricanes because it destroys people, our most important resource.'[4] Aggravating this is the fact that any unprovided-for loss of human resources has a particularly severe impact in territories with small populations, as in the case of many of the island states where there would be difficulty in making good the premature or unanticipated loss of even one strategically placed individual.

Studies by the Caribbean Epidemiology Centre (CAREC) and the University of the West Indies (UWI) suggest that the economic impact of HIV/AIDS is likely to be considerable in a number of countries. The studies estimate that if current trends continue the epidemic could cost Jamaica 6.2 per cent of its national income in the period 2000-2005; the cost to St. Lucia for the same period could be 4.7 per cent, and to Trinidad and Tobago 4.2 per cent (Theodore, 2000). For both Jamaica and Trinidad and Tobago, the estimate is that HIV/AIDS alone would cost more than twice the public sector allocation to the health sector and almost as much as what each of these countries spends annually on health care. The Caribbean Task Force on HIV/AIDS has adopted 5 per cent as being indicative of the GDP loss that the epidemic will occasion for countries across the region. This is almost the equivalent of the entire regional spending on health care, since on the average countries in the region allocate between 5 and 6 per cent of their national income to health services.

The epidemic could affect the tourist-dependent economies of many Caribbean territories in various ways, by deterring tourists, reducing the ability to offer services, and increasing vulnerability to infection. The sensitivity of these economies to external shocks became evident in the significant drop in tourist revenues following the terrorist attacks on New York in September 2001. HIV/AIDS could provide another such shock. But it must also be borne in mind that tourism tends to be associated with an increasingly active commercial sex industry, with the implications this has for the increased transmission of HIV infection within the region.

Because most of those affected by HIV/AIDS are in their most productive years economically – at the end of 1998, 83 per cent of the reported cases in the Caribbean were in the age group 15 to 54 years and 50 per cent in the group aged 25 to 34 years – the loss of productive adults could have extensive negative impacts on economic sectors other than tourism, as for example on agriculture, mining, timber, finance and trade (World Bank, 2000: 19). The negative consequences would be due principally to the loss of productivity arising from absenteeism, sickness, deaths, and the replacement of skilled individuals by those with less expertise, and from the increased costs associated with medical care, the premature payment of terminal benefits, and the recruitment and training of replacement labour. A further major concern is the way the epidemic leads to the loss of social capital, eroding the social structure of communities, undermining the capacity of governments to provide basic social services, and affecting their ability to provide the enabling environment of efficient economic management, regulation and legal frameworks so necessary for development.

Another effect that has been identified is the potential of the epidemic to lead to increased insecurity and instability. The security implications of the disease were highlighted by the attention given to the epidemic by the United Nations Security Council in January 2000, the first time it ever considered a health issue (this being the way HIV/AIDS was mostly considered at that time). The many interactions of Caribbean countries with other countries in the western hemisphere, especially those in North America, draw attention to sensitivities and concerns that the Caribbean could provide a route by which the disease might extend its grip in the United States and Canada. The United States, in particular, shows deep concern about the security dimensions of the disease arising from the way it can undermine economic growth, exacerbate social tensions, diminish military preparedness, create huge social welfare costs, and weaken already beleaguered states. The early history of the disease in the Caribbean and the stigma to which Haitians visiting North America were exposed are indications of the way the situation could develop.

Accentuating the implications for security and international relations is the fact that the second highest urban HIV prevalence in the United States occurs in San Juan, the capital of Puerto Rico, which is a self-governing Commonwealth of the United States. Unlike other severely affected parts of the Caribbean, HIV transmission in Puerto Rico is strongly associated with injecting drug use.

Confidentiality

A unique challenge faced by the Caribbean in responding to HIV/ AIDS is that of ensuring that confidentiality is respected at all times, particularly in services that address the needs of young people. Confidentiality poses special problems for small island communities where the close and warm interactions that sustain communities may also lead to extensive sharing about one another's affairs (*Box 3*). It is significant that in 1996 recommendations from a task force to the Caribbean Conference of Ministers Responsible for Health included a recommendation reiterating the importance of confidentiality and advising that those who breach it should be disciplined, a recommendation that the ministers accepted (Walrond, 2000: 63). Young people will not use health and voluntary counselling (VCT) services if they fear that confidential information may be divulged to their families, employers, or members of the community. In relation to the silence and stigma that is attached to HIV/AIDS, the aim should be to break down the walls and bring it out into the open. In relation to what transpires in health and VCT sessions, the objective should be to strengthen the walls of confidentiality and silence so that clients who use such services will feel protected.

Box 3. The challenge of confidentiality in the Caribbean

Throughout the Caribbean, the population's inability to deal with confidentiality has impacted heavily on the PLAs…. It is alleged that the majority of breaches (of confidentiality) occur at public health and social support institutions…. Health care workers and clerical officers are the ones who tell friends and relatives about who is infected, especially in the smaller territories. This has hampered the development of organised support services including hotlines. Most persons contend that each country in the region is so small that everyone knows everyone else so there is constant fear of disclosure even in a therapeutic environment (Francis, 2000: 194).

'If you had a problem and you talked to somebody outside of the home, for example, a guidance counsellor or another relative, and they in turn spoke to your parents, you usually got into more trouble with your parents afterwards – they might even beat you for taking your family business outside' (Dunn, 2002: 37).

'I do not use any of the HIV services because it is not confidential and I don't like that. This is a small island and people talk about your business [HIV positive status] and I do not want to get cut off' (Dicks, 2001: 79).

The regional response to HIV/AIDS in the Caribbean

Ministries of Health in the Caribbean were aware for a long time that HIV/AIDS constituted a major and growing problem for the region. Initially, the epidemic was regarded principally as a health concern and did not receive the high profile it deserved as 'the most formidable development challenge of our time' (Kofi Annan, UN Secretary-General). Almost every country established its own National AIDS Programme (NAP), but the scope and the effectiveness of the response varied considerably. In almost every case the NAP was firmly anchored in the country's Ministry of Health, a situation that is beginning to show signs of changing. Barbados is the first Caribbean country where the programme is now housed in the Office of the Prime Minister. A few other countries are starting to follow the Barbadian lead.

In many instances the National AIDS Programmes were not equipped with the requisite capacity to ensure that the epidemic was addressed in a comprehensive and effective way. In a number of countries, adjustments to the economic shocks of the 1980s and early 1990s and rising levels of debt meant that resources for dealing with the epidemic, even from the limited perspective of its being principally a health concern, were inadequate. In particular, the region experienced difficulty in developing the qualified human resources needed to guide and implement an effective response.

However, the period spanning the end of the twentieth century and the beginning of the twenty-first, saw the initiation of more holistic regional and national responses. The catalyst was provided by a series of high-level meetings of heads of state and leaders of government throughout the region. These ushered in a new era of public awareness, HIV/AIDS visibility, and political commitment to confront the epidemic in all its manifestations. Immediate outcomes of this new regional resolve were the development of the Caribbean Regional Strategic Plan of Action for HIV/AIDS (CRSPAH), the establishment of the Pan-Caribbean Partnership Against AIDS (PANCAP), and commitments to strengthen the capacity of regional institutions to plan, coordinate, implement and monitor a region-wide response to the epidemic. Another outcome was the increased international commitment to help Caribbean institutions and countries galvanize their response to the epidemic. Notable among these has been assistance from the European Union to enhance the capacity of a number of regional institutions to respond to HIV/AIDS needs, and the approval by the World Bank of a US$155 million dollar multi-country HIV/AIDS prevention and control-lending programme.[5]

Working with a broad array of partners and National AIDS Programmes, the UNAIDS Caribbean office is a leading advocate for regional action against the epidemic. Among its co-sponsors, PAHO/WHO seeks to bolster the response of the health sector to the epidemic through efforts concentrated on the strengthening of health systems, the prevention of infection, the provision of care and support, and the mitigation of the impact of the illness on individuals and communities. A major focus for UNICEF in the region is the CARICOM-led regional Health and Family Life Education (HFLE) initiative. UNDP, as the main coordinator of United Nations activities for development at country level, continues to explore ways of confronting the development impact and consequences of the epidemic. Of special relevance to this book is the significant headway that has been registered by UNESCO in addressing both regional and national AIDS – and education issues. In recent years, its Caribbean office has become increasingly involved in advocacy, partnership building, capacity building, strategy development and targeted fundraising for HIV/AIDS-related activities.

Notwithstanding this progress, the epidemic continues to spiral upwards at national and regional levels with the exception of the Bahamas and, more recently, Haiti. Further moves needed in the region are the development of national-level plans that take account of the principles formulated in the regional strategic plan for HIV/AIDS, more purposeful coordination on the part of donors and the UNAIDS co-sponsors, a clarification of roles and responsibilities, the disentanglement of HIV/AIDS from the health sector, and greater assurance in facing the sensitive issues of sex tourism, the commercial sex industry, men who have sex with men, and the early age of sexual activity. There is also room for the region to learn more from what has been happening elsewhere, especially in sub-Saharan Africa and South-East Asia. In many respects, the region still awaits a comprehensive, dynamic, and wide-ranging response to the epidemic. The education sector in the region has the potential to provide the leadership in spearheading this response.

Notes

1.   The HDI is a measure of human development in a country as manifested by the prospects for a long and healthy life (life expectancy at birth), knowledge (adult literacy rate and combined primary, secondary and tertiary enrolment rates), and a decent standard of living (real GDP per capita). When combined in a predetermined way, the variables shown in brackets lead to the HDI. This index is always less than one. In 1999, the HDI for 162 countries ranged from 0.939 (Norway) to 0.258 (Sierra Leone).

2.   The OECS consists of the Leeward Islands (British Virgin Islands, Anguilla, St. Kitts and Nevis, Antigua and Barbuda, and Montserrat) and the Windward Islands (Dominica, St. Lucia, St. Vincent and the Grenadines, and Grenada).

3.   UNAIDS classifies an epidemic as being low level when HIV prevalence does not consistently exceed five percent in any defined sub-population; as being concentrated when HIV prevalence consistently exceeds five percent in at least one defined subpopulation but remains below one percent in pregnant women in urban areas; and as being generalized when HIV prevalence consistently exceeds one percent in pregnant women nation-wide.

4.   Atherton Martin, Minister of Planning, Dominica, in a statement at the closing meeting of the Caribbean Consultative Group for Economic Development, Washington DC, 12 June 2000.

5.   At the time of writing, this facility had been used to finance loans of US$25 million to the Dominican Republic, US$15.5 million to Barbados, US$15 million to Jamaica, US$20 million to Trinidad and Tobago, and US$6 million to Grenada, to support their National AIDS Programmes.

HIV/AIDS AND EDUCATION

CHAPTER 3

Education and HIV/AIDS: Global Lessons

There is a two-way interaction between education and HIV/AIDS. As a result of its impact on various facets of the education sector, the epidemic can undermine the potential of the sector to deliver education of adequate quality to young people and other beneficiaries. On the other hand, through its effect on various facets of the epidemic, education can contribute significantly to the prevention of HIV transmission, the care and support of those infected or affected by the disease, and the mitigation of the epidemic's negative impacts.

In view of this, the approach of the education sector in dealing with the epidemic should be guided by two principles that operate simultaneously:

- minimise the impact of HIV/AIDS on education;
- maximise the impact of education on HIV/AIDS in the areas of prevention, care and support, and the management and alleviation of impacts.

What HIV/AIDS can do to education

'What HIV/AIDS does to the human body, it also does to institutions. It undermines those institutions that protect us' (Piot, 2000). The truth of this can be seen by comparing what HIV does to the human body and what it does to a system, such as an educational system, or to a major institution, such as a school or a university.

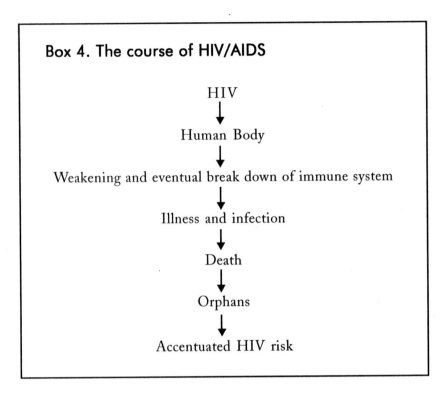

Box 4. The course of HIV/AIDS

HIV

Human Body

Weakening and eventual break down of immune system

Illness and infection

Death

Orphans

Accentuated HIV risk

When a person is infected with the human immuno-deficiency virus (HIV), the body's immune system weakens and eventually breaks down (*Box 4*). This leaves the individual prey to the hazards of a multitude of infections and certain types of cancer. In the absence of the costly antiretroviral therapy that can suppress HIV activity, the infected individual will in all likelihood eventually succumb to the serious cluster of illnesses that define AIDS. When infected adults die, they very frequently leave orphans behind. For the adult, life has ended. For the orphan the tragedy continues and may even worsen, since orphaned children are more vulnerable than other children to HIV infection (Mugabe, Stirling and Whiteside, 2002).

In a similar way, in the absence of appropriate measures, the education system in a country that is seriously affected by HIV/AIDS is also in danger of being weakened and disrupted. The epidemic greatly increases the scale of existing educational problems.

Box 5. The impact of HIV/AIDS on the education system

HIV

↓

Education system

↓

Weakening and disruption of system

↓

Increased scale of existing problems
within the education sector

↓

Reactive changes, adjustments, innovations

↓

Education sector turbulence

↓

Inability to deliver educational services

This in turn leads to a number of reactive changes and adaptations, considerable turbulence within the sector, and the possibility of its not being able to deliver its mandated services (*Box 5*). Critical tasks for policy-makers and planners in education are to identify the potential areas of impact and to design appropriate responses. Some interventions may take place in reaction to circumstances that have actually been experienced. However, coping with the HIV/AIDS situation in the education sector requires more than this. There is need to be proactive, anticipating what might possibly happen, forestalling undesirable situations, and managing the circumstances with three objectives in mind: (1) enabling the education system to pursue and attain its essential goals; (2) using the sector's potential to slow down the rate of new infections; and (3) providing care and support for infected and affected learners and educators.

Essentially, educational institutions and programmes seek to establish arrangements that try to ensure that learners learn and educators teach in an environment that supports learning. In countries affected by the epidemic, HIV/AIDS has an increasingly negative impact on these three major areas – it affects learners, educators and the learning environment. The impact in these areas may be sufficient to make learning difficult or even impossible, impede teaching, and create an environment that is not conducive to the provision of good quality education. Furthermore, the epidemic has progressive major financial implications for the education sector and can have a significant negative impact on educational management and planning.

The potential impact of HIV/AIDS on learners

The principal beneficiaries of an education programme or system are young people, ranging in age from infancy to young adulthood. It is mostly the young who are in schools, colleges and universities, developing the values, attitudes, knowledge and skills that will serve them subsequently in adult life. It is also largely the also young who participate in out-of-school and non-formal education and training programmes.

But if education is largely the sphere of the young, so also is HIV/AIDS. As noted already in *Chapter 1*, young people constitute about one-third of those infected with HIV and AIDS. In addition, countless young people are living with the disease in their families and the communities on which they depend for their psycho-social and economic support. These situations can affect the school and institutional learning of young people, leading to non-participation, irregular participation, and participation that is not conducive to good learning.

In the countries that are hardest hit by HIV/AIDS, school-aged children from households with persons who are in the late stages of HIV/AIDS may not attend school at all and many young people and adults may fail to participate in educational programmes designed to meet their needs. This occurs because:

- By reducing or making new demands on resources, AIDS in the family makes it difficult for the potential learners to meet the costs associated with their schooling or educational programmes.

- Those who should be attending school or participating in an educational programme must work in their homes or in family income-generating activities, to replace those who are sick or have died.

- Those who should be learning must look after the sick in their homes or take on the tasks of others who are looking after the sick.

- There is little home pressure or interest in school attendance or educational programme participation because of perceptions that the learner may have only a short life and hence could make better use of the time available.

- Those who should be learners may have become members of child-headed households where either there is nobody to ensure that they attend school or they must work to generate the resources needed for survival.

In almost all of these situations, girls tend to be more seriously affected than boys. Hence, HIV/AIDS has especially adverse effects on the education of girls. Specifically, it makes it more difficult to ensure the attainment of the EFA goals of the universalization of school education for girls and the closing of the gender gap at the primary and secondary education levels (and a fortiori at the tertiary level).

Again, in countries hardest hit by HIV/AIDS, the school attendance of many learners can be erratic for several reasons. These may include periodic household demands for the child's services arising from the sickness of a household member; the child's own illness, which may be recurrent and compounded by poverty and inability to obtain medication; and death in the family or local community, followed by funeral attendance and periods of mourning. The participation of learners in non-school-based programmes can be affected in the same ways. Once again girls tend to be more seriously affected than boys and this means that they will not complete their education cycle or programme.

Third, the learning of those who actually attend school or participate in educational programmes may be impeded by the following factors:

- the trauma arising from the experience of seeing a parent or other loved adult enduring remorseless suffering and a dehumanizing death;

- the psychological distress of seeing a teacher or fellow-learner experiencing the devastating effects of AIDS;

- the sense of fear, isolation, prejudice and discrimination suffered by learners coming from households where there is a person suffering from AIDS or which have experienced an AIDS death. Reports from countries in various parts of the world speak of the petty taunting and derision that such learners may experience;

- in high-prevalence countries, there is a pervasive atmosphere of illness and death that subtly intrudes itself into the lives of schools and other educational institutions;

- the disruption of teaching and learning activities caused by irregular teacher schedules, funeral attendance, personal concerns, resource limitations, and other HIV-related circumstances (see below).

The potential impact of HIV/AIDS on educators

The potential impact of HIV/AIDS on educators is experienced through deaths, sickness, absenteeism, workload effects, and levels of morale.

'While many countries lack reliable data on AIDS-related deaths and HIV prevalence among teachers, evidence points to an increased teacher mortality rate in the presence of HIV/AIDS' (World Bank, 2002: 11). While the increased mortality rate may be similar to that in the general population, its occurrence deprives the profession of teachers and other staff who, in other circumstances, would have put their qualifications and experience at the service of education for several more years. Moreover, in addition to mortality losses, education and training systems suffer the loss of qualified personnel to areas where HIV/AIDS-occasioned needs are emerging.

Teacher attrition has always been a running sore for the sector in countries where teachers are not fully satisfied with their conditions and terms of service. In recent years, the active recruitment of English-speaking teachers has compounded the drift of teachers from the Commonwealth Caribbean to North America. But the Caribbean and other severely affected HIV/AIDS regions could also begin to share the experience of sub-Saharan Africa where the epidemic has created an additional pull of teachers away from schools, as other sectors of government, business, and industry seek to fill positions left vacant by AIDS-related deaths.

Teachers who die or withdraw permanently from teaching have to be replaced – if a replacement is available. Occasionally it may be possible to find a temporary replacement among retired teachers – a strategy to which some severely affected countries are having increasing recourse. The more commonly adopted strategy is to wait for the annual output from the teacher training institutions and in the meantime either to seek the services of an unqualified teacher or to do without – spreading the load among others in the school.

There is a limit to the applicability of this strategy. Training programmes are not usually planned in such a way as to flood the market with teachers surplus to requirements. Instead they usually seek to produce enough qualified teachers to cover projected retirements, some expansion or contraction of the educational system, and general loss due to known rates of mortality and occupational mobility.

Increased teacher mortality due to AIDS may raise the demand for new college graduates (whose numbers may also have declined because of AIDS-related illness and death among trainees) above the supply. This may necessitate that affected schools continue their dependence on unqualified teachers or function with fewer teachers.

In the hardest hit countries of sub-Saharan Africa, ad hoc efforts have been made to provide services when staffing falls below the approved norms. Some insufficiently staffed schools have had to combine grades at the same level into a single class or introduce forms of multigrade teaching. Collapsing classes may mean that class sizes become so large that student learning is jeopardised. Multigrade teaching can be an excellent approach where enrolments are low, teachers are acquainted with the methodology, and the necessary resources are forthcoming. It is understandable that it may be adopted as an emergency response to understaffing in some situations. But if class sizes are average to large, where teachers have received no special training in this approach, where no resources have been set aside, the prolonged adoption of multigrade teaching is not likely to promote optimal student learning. Although neither approach provides a permanent or desirable solution, education officials in countries where HIV/AIDS is a major problem are aware that it is by adopting practices like these that many schools actually continue to operate.

Officials face staffing problems of a different nature when AIDS (or some other cause) leads to the death of the sole teacher in a small rural school. The transfer of a teacher from another school may not be possible – there may be nobody suitable, the needs of other schools may not allow the release of one of their teachers, or a teacher may refuse to be transferred to the teacherless school because of fear that it remains 'haunted' by HIV/AIDS. This last possibility highlights a consideration that always needs to be borne in mind, that notwithstanding their specialised knowledge and training, teachers in common with other members of the general population share many common misapprehensions about the disease.

At higher levels of the education system, the numerical losses due to AIDS are further complicated by losses in specialised areas. The loss of a general educator is serious for any institution or programme, but provision can sometimes be made by redeploying another teacher or enlarging classes. This becomes more difficult when the loss is that of a secondary school teacher in hard-to-staff areas, such as mathematics or physics, or of a tertiary level lecturer in a highly specialised vocational or academic subject, such as metalwork or management accounting. Faced with losses of this kind, institutions and systems might no longer be able to offer important programmes and might have to discontinue certain subject areas, unless preparations were made for such an eventuality by training directed at widening the expertise base of existing staff.

The progressive nature of HIV/AIDS leads to teachers and other educators either attending irregularly or being absent from their post for several months prior to their final AIDS-related sickness. It is currently accepted that the sickness of AIDS is likely to evolve over a period of ten years, during which time the infected person may be absent because of recurring illnesses for a total of 260 days (World Bank, 2002: 41). This situation has two negative outcomes for education. First, there is reduced educator productivity, whether this is in the area of actual teaching or of some other educational activity, such as curriculum, research, examinations, management, planning, or financial accounts work. In the classroom, the immediate effect is the haphazard or random delivery of lessons and an almost inevitable failure by the majority of learners to make the progress they should. Second, in almost all cases the infected educators remain on the payroll, thereby tying down funds that might otherwise have been used for the employment of substitute or replacement staff. In addition, even when physically present in the classroom or on duty, the infected educator may experience a level of disengagement with, and detachment from, the teaching or other task that would impair effective teaching (Badcock-Walters, 2002).

In hard-hit areas, two other AIDS-related factors lead to increased absenteeism on the part of healthy teachers, other educators and workers throughout the entire workforce – caring for sick relatives at home and attending funerals. Since the burden of care falls mostly on women, female educators and office staff frequently find themselves pulled between three competing roles, that of their professional work area, that of managing a household, and that of attending to sick persons who require almost round-the-clock care. In this context it is important to note that a serious gap in current policy development in response to HIV/AIDS in the education sector is the failure to take account of the disproportionate impacts the disease makes on female educators, and the need to make flexible arrangements that will allow them to harmonise in a satisfactory way the responsibilities arising from their three roles.

In many cultures there are strong expectations regarding funeral attendance and participation in the rites that lead up to burial or cremation. The pressures arising from the frequency of death that characterises the AIDS crisis are slowly transforming these traditions so that less imposition is placed on the resources of the bereaved family and on the time of funeral participants. Nevertheless, educational institutions, business concerns and government offices continue to experience considerable absenteeism because of funeral attendance. In some countries, funerals occur mostly at weekends so that they cause minimal disruption of normal operations but in others they occur throughout the week. In such circumstances, a class may have to go without a teacher for a few days at a time. In a study carried out across a number of HIV/AIDS-affected countries, it was found that absenteeism due to funeral attendance accounted for six per cent of the increased labour costs due to HIV/AIDS (Whiteside and Sunter, 2000: 101). It could well be that funeral attendance reduces the productivity of educational institutions by at least a similar amount.

HIV/AIDS also makes diverse impacts that tend to increase a teacher's responsibilities and workload:

- teachers may have to take on additional responsibilities to cover for a sick or absent colleague;
- teachers may be required to teach in areas where they are not expert because the experts are sick or have died;
- teachers are increasingly being asked to integrate HIV/AIDS considerations into their classroom work, but many do not feel competent to do so;
- the teaching of life-skills has become integral to the curriculum for education in an AIDS-infected society, but many teachers are not conversant with the methods or approaches needed for effective teaching in this area;

- teachers face new demands because of the behavioural, emotional and psychological problems brought into the classroom by infected and affected learners;

- many teachers find that in addition to their teaching work they are also expected to provide counselling services for affected or infected learners;

- leisure time is being eroded through an increasing number of workshops and in-service training activities designed to make teachers knowledgeable and competent in HIV-related areas.

In addition, among teachers in high-prevalence countries, the frequent experience of death and serious sickness in their families, communities and schools tends to undermine their morale. The situation is aggravated when teachers see their incomes eroded through the re-direction of their resources to medical and funeral expenses and sometimes to local fund-raising ventures for the support of orphans and other vulnerable children. There is also an underlying sense of uneasiness and fear arising from what they observe around them, from concern lest they too may be HIV infected, from the misconception that HIV is necessarily fatal, and from a sense of fatalistic hopelessness about the value of HIV testing when there is little prospect of effective treatment for those found to be infected. Many yearn to know about their HIV status. Most fear the diagnosis.

The potential impact of HIV/AIDS on educational provision and outcomes

HIV/AIDS can make significant impacts on educational provision and outcomes by its potential to affect three critical dimensions: costs and financing, national educational planning and sector management and quality.

The epidemic has potential adverse *financial implications* for education because of the way it affects the availability of resources and increases costs:

1.   HIV/AIDS affects the availability of resources for education because:

- households are less well able to support education, owing to AIDS-occasioned reductions in family incomes, the diversion of family resources to medical care, and increasing outlays in response to the needs of orphans and vulnerable children;

- the ability of communities to contribute labour or other resources for school development is reduced because of the way AIDS weakens a community's productive capacity, necessitates heavy medical, mourning and funeral expenses, and increases demands on a community's time and work capacity because of the loss of active community members;

- the ability of the private sector to support educational development is impaired, owing to the way HIV/AIDS reduces its profitability by lowering productivity, increasing costs, diverting productive resources, and affecting the market for business products;

- public funds for education are less than they would be in a non-AIDS situation, owing to the AIDS-related slowing down in the growth of national income and to the need to make larger allocations for health and AIDS-related interventions.

2.   HIV/AIDS increases the costs of educational provision because:

- additional educators must be trained to replace those lost to the disease;

- death benefits, which will be greater than those payable subsequent to retirement, must be paid on behalf of those who die while still in active service;

- the introduction of HIV preventive education within the curriculum, and the consequent development, production and dissemination of textbooks and learning materials, necessitate additional expenditure;

- additional in-service programmes have to be introduced to equip teachers in the broad field of HIV/AIDS education;

- HIV/AIDS has to be built into programmes for initial and ongoing teacher preparation, and educators have to be retrained for this purpose;

- mainstreaming HIV/AIDS into the management and administrative functions of an education ministry entails additional cost;

- provision must be made for more extensive access to psycho-social counselling for HIV/AIDS-affected educators and learners;

- incentives must be provided to stimulate orphans and other children affected by HIV/AIDS to participate in school or other educational programmes.

The estimated scale of the additional costs is staggeringly high. The EFA Monitoring Report, published towards the end of 2002, estimated that in 46 developing countries HIV/AIDS would add an additional US$975 million per year to the costs of achieving universal primary education. The report notes that the 'cost implications of HIV/AIDS are so extensive and so pervasive that they may serve better than anything else to demonstrate the urgency of protecting the education sector against the ravages of the epidemic and of using the potential of education to extend greater protection to society' (UNESCO, 2002: 22).

HIV/AIDS affects the *planning and management* of an education system because of:

- the overriding need to manage the system to promote the prevention of HIV transmission, the care and support of infected and affected educators and learners, and the reduction of impacts;

- loss through mortality and sickness of various education officials charged with responsibility for planning, implementing, and managing policies, programmes and projects;

- the need for evidence-based information that brings to the fore the current and likely future impact of the epidemic on learners, educators, institutions, and the system itself (impact assessments);

- the need for all capacity-building and human resource planning to provide for:

  (a) potential personnel losses,

    (b) developing new approaches, knowledge, skills and attitudes that will enable the system to cope with the epidemic's impacts and monitor how it is doing so, and

    (c) establishing intra-sectoral epidemic-related information systems.

- the need for more accountable and cost-effective financial management at all levels in response to reduced national, community and private resources for education;

- the need for sensitive care in dealing with personnel and the human rights issues of AIDS-affected employees and their dependants;

- the need for a sector-wide strategic approach that will spell out how the education ministry intends to address HIV/AIDS.

HIV/AIDS does not incapacitate or remove large numbers of individuals all at once. Instead it whittles away steadily at the human resource base. Because of this, the need for management adjustment to many of the potential impacts of HIV/AIDS is not always immediately apparent. Education authorities in low or medium-prevalence countries may not see that their systems are at risk, whereas all the time, because of its insidious nature, the disease is relentlessly eroding overall systemic capacity. In view of this, even in low or medium-prevalence countries, policy-makers and educational planners will do well to examine what is happening in their respective systems and to pre-empt disruptive HIV/AIDS impacts by making the necessary proactive adjustments.

It is largely through its planning and management structures that an education ministry will coordinate and direct its response to the epidemic. A critical task will be to protect its core functions. Hence it must use its planning and management structures to ensure that faced with the actual and potential ravages of the epidemic, the education system continues to function in a satisfactory way. The criterion for success will be the system's ability to maintain its productivity and continue to provide meaningful and relevant educational services. In practice, this will mean that despite the presence of the epidemic, the system works so that teachers are teaching, children are enrolling and staying in school, older learners are learning, managers are managing, and personnel, finance and professional development systems are performing adequately.

But in the circumstances of HIV/AIDS, 'business as usual' is never an adequate response. The education sector's planning and management structures must also be used to further HIV prevention, promote care and support for infected and affected educators and learners, mitigate the institutional impacts of the epidemic, and respond creatively and flexibly to its new and ever more complex challenges. These issues are further explored in *Chapter 7*.

Most educators would agree that *quality in education* implies (1) efficiency in meeting set goals, (2) relevance to human and environmental needs and conditions, and (3) 'something more' in relation to the pursuit of excellence and human betterment (Hawes and Stephens, 1990: 11). One touchstone of quality so defined is learning achievement.

In an environment that is heavily dominated by HIV/AIDS, learning achievement is likely to be inhibited by such factors as:

- frequent absenteeism of individual teachers or tutors, due to repeated bouts of sickness, care for the sick at home, or funeral attendance;
- shortages of qualified educators and increased reliance on those who are less well qualified or experienced;
- the cessation of learning activities (particularly if the school is small) – periodically, because of teacher sickness; for a longer period, if a teacher dies;
- lethargy and a sense of fatalism in teachers and tutors who know that they have HIV or AIDS;
- teacher uneasiness and uncertainty about personal HIV status;
- frequent student absence due to the need to care for the sick at home;
- intermittent student participation, with an irregular start-stop, 'drop out/drop in' pattern;

- repeated occasions for grief and mourning in the school or training institution, in families, and in the community;
- difficulty on the part of both educator and learner in concentrating on teaching and learning activities because of concern for those who are sick at home;
- unhappiness and fear of stigmatization and ostracism on the part of both teachers and learners who have been affected by HIV/AIDS;
- uncertainty and distrust in the relations between learners and teachers (who may be caricatured as abusers of children or as those responsible for HIV introduction and spread).

The combination of HIV/AIDS-related random teaching and learning, the loss of educators, low teacher and learner morale, reduced financial resources, and inadequate management provision all reduce an education system's ability to meet set educational goals. It is difficult to maintain relevance to the human and environmental situation, and ensure the extra dimensions of creativity, stimulation, excitement, concern for others, and happiness that bespeak quality and excellence in education. Thus the epidemic comprehensively jeopardises the attainment of the EFA goal of improving all aspects of the quality of education.

Vulnerability factors inherent to the education sector

The HIV/AIDS epidemic is so all-encompassing that it raises many difficult questions. One relates to the way the education sector itself is organised and operates. The pervasiveness of the effects makes it necessary to ask whether the sector itself may provide an environment that increases vulnerability to HIV. Major impacts of the epidemic are the explosion in the scale of existing systemic and management problems in education, and making dysfunctional systems worse. But in addition, education systems in various parts of the world have inherent policy and operational features that either heighten the possibility that individuals might engage in behaviour that could put them at risk of HIV infection, or prevent the system itself from responding in an adaptable way to the impacts of the epidemic.

For individuals, the education sector may unwittingly establish potentially high-risk HIV situations through policies and procedures governing such areas as:

- *School arrangements*: A large proportion of those attending primary school are already sexually active (*Figure 2*), but in general schools at this level do little to help learners develop behaviour patterns for the responsible management of their sexuality. In addition, many learners are in danger of sexual harassment from their peers, strangers, and possibly even school personnel (Kelly, 2000). Learners who are required by circumstances (or parental wishes) to stay in school hostels merit special consideration. Providing term-time hostel accommodation for young, sexually active learners who receive almost no comprehensive guidance or support increases the risk that they will engage in sexual activity with each another or with individuals from the surrounding community. This may be aggravated by the fact that primary school children and adolescents rarely communicate with their parents or other adults about sexual and reproductive health issues, but rely greatly on information – some of it false or misleading – acquired casually or from their peers.

- *Teacher deployment*: The practice of requiring trainee teachers who are posted to a school for practice teaching to make their own temporary accommodation arrangements may place them in situations of personal risk. The same goes for teachers who are posted to schools, away from their families and with inadequate initial arrangements for their accommodation. The absence of family, loneliness, and the availability of some money combine to make such individuals vulnerable to casual sex (or quasi-steady temporary relationships) and HIV infection.

There are also features of the education system that have become so firmly entrenched that they do not respond readily to the demands and impacts of HIV/AIDS. Instances include:

- The strong teacher-centred classroom approach that experiences difficulty in accommodating the highly interactive learner-centred and peer-to-peer approach which meaningful HIV/AIDS education requires.

- The predominance of the cognitive, academic approach in school learning, accompanied by considerable downgrading of concern for the psycho-social, moral and practical development of learners.

In terms of UNESCO's four pillars of learning, the major concern is with 'learning to know' (UNESCO, 1996). Systems give much less attention to 'learning to do', 'learning to be' and 'learning to live together', types of learning which are fundamental to a comprehensive response to HIV/AIDS.

- Education systems tend not to take responsibility for those who are not enrolled in their institutions. Notwithstanding structural efforts to expand systems and compel attendance, a number of young people are not reached by the formal educational system. Others drop out at various ages, many of them before they have acquired a sufficient repertoire of knowledge, skills and values to serve them through life. In the situation of HIV/AIDS, education systems should feel duty bound to assume some responsibility to enable these young people live safe and productive lives.

- The allocation of secondary and service roles to women and girls in ways that enhance the perception that it is right and natural for females to minister to the needs of males. This can be seen in circumstances that vary from de facto limitations on the fields of study undertaken by women and girls to the practice of assuming that secretarial, catering and cleaning responsibilities should automatically be entrusted to girls and women.

The enumeration of these points suggests that HIV/AIDS demands that education ministries radically reexamine their policies, procedures and modes of operation. Where prevalence rates are high, ministries can no longer carry on with business as usual. The epidemic puts the entire organizational culture under the spotlight, challenges many of its basic assumptions, and necessitates a fundamental questioning of virtually sacrosanct understandings and approaches.

What education can do to HIV/AIDS

The report of the Dakar World Education Forum states that 'education can be a powerful force – perhaps the most powerful force of all – in combating the spread of HIV/AIDS' (UNESCO, 2000: 22-23). The forum had sound reasons for its affirmation. HIV/AIDS has no cure. A vaccine is only dimly coming into sight. High costs, the fragility of medical infrastructures, adverse side effects, and concerns about its continued effectiveness suggest that antiretroviral therapy will never provide a complete solution. In these circumstances, humankind's only mechanism for dealing with the epidemic is education. It is a necessary mechanism and a potent mechanism:

1. Education is necessary for galvanising the political momentum and community mobilization that are central to success against HIV/AIDS.

2. Education is necessary for reducing stigma and discrimination – twin pillars that support the continued spread of the disease and undercut care and support for the infected and affected.

3. Education enters in a fundamental way into every communication on prevention.

4. Some form of education is intrinsic to every programme of treatment and care.

5. Formal school education and non-formal programmes for young people reach into communities and families in ways that no other services do.

6. Formal and non-formal education programmes are largely the province of the young, the category at greatest risk of becoming infected with HIV.

7. There is a growing body of evidence that education empowers individuals to take decisions that are more life-affirming. In this sense, the more education, the less likelihood of HIV.

Early evidence from severely affected countries showed a tendency for levels of HIV infection to be higher among those who were better educated and more affluent. But this evidence for a positive relationship between level of education and HIV prevalence derives from individuals who had become sexually active in the comparatively early stages of the epidemic when the behavioural correlates of infection were less well understood and less widely disseminated. Many individuals in this group continue to suffer extensive morbidity and mortality. More recent evidence, however, shows a distinct change in the relationship, with more educated younger people emerging as less likely to be HIV infected (*Figure 3*, Vandermoortele and Delamonica, 2000). In other words, it is now becoming clearer that education does help individuals protect themselves against HIV infection. The school *is* an institution that protects.

Figure 3. The changing relationship between HIV prevalence and level of education

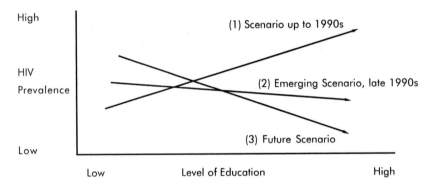

Education works against HIV/AIDS in a number of ways. Most fundamentally, there seems to be something inherent in the very process of becoming educated that equips individuals with the capabilities they need to keep themselves HIV free. The very fact of being educated, of having attended school for a certain number of years, appears to be fundamental. Initiation into a learning culture, orientation to a possible and desirable better future, and the acquisition of basic literacy and numeracy skills, seem to be key ingredients. But these apart, it does not seem to be so much how one has learned or even what one has learned that matters. What counts is *that* one has learned.

But what is learned and how it is learned can greatly enhance the potency of education to work against HIV/AIDS, preventing its transmission, caring for and supporting those infected or affected, and mitigating its impacts. This is because good education is about:

- *Learning to know*: it communicates comprehensive and accurate information about the disease;

- *Learning to do*: it fosters the acquisition of psycho-social and other skills that enhance the ability to protect oneself against infection;

- *Learning to live together*: it promotes a compassionate, caring, rights-based, non-judgmental approach to every person, irrespective of HIV status;

- *Learning to be*: it supports the development of life-affirming attitudes, skills and value systems that help learners make healthy life choices, resist negative pressures, and minimise harmful behaviours (cf. UNESCO, 1996: 85-97).

Limitations in the educational approaches adopted

To date, education ministries, confronted with the need to take urgent action against HIV/AIDS, have responded by adopting a predominantly curriculum-based approach. Clearly, curriculum concerns, and all that they imply in terms of structure, training, teaching, learning and educational materials, are the core responsibilities of an education ministry. By responding to HIV/AIDS in terms of the curriculum, education ministries were working in the area they knew best and in which they were the acknowledged experts. However, curriculum messages relating to HIV/AIDS tended to be based on models that did not take sufficient account of wide contextual factors. As was the case elsewhere in the world, early generations of school programmes to prevent HIV/AIDS operated on the premiss that providing knowledge would meet the need (Schenker, 2001). With their strong focus on an information-driven rational approach, these early HIV/AIDS curricula did not pay adequate attention to the social context, and largely overlooked the affective, emotional domain (*Chapter 1*). In addition, the curriculum response to HIV/AIDS seldom capitalised on local cultures. The perspectives of western bio-medical and behavioural sciences dominated, at the expense of those based on traditional beliefs and understandings.

There can be no doubt about the need for young people to be better informed and know the facts about HIV/AIDS, and education programmes must ensure that this is done. The challenge to education to do so has been highlighted by information coming from national surveys that reveal an astonishing lack of knowledge about AIDS, HIV transmission, prevention and sexuality among the young people surveyed (UNAIDS/UNICEF/WHO, 2002).

A first essential is to ensure the beneficiaries of education systems know all the facts. But the facts alone will not save people from infection. Creating awareness does not necessarily lead to the adoption or maintenance of life-enhancing behaviour. Evidence from school-based HIV prevention programmes bears eloquent testimony to this (Bennell, Hyde and Swainson, 2002). What is needed in addition is to help young people adopt the attitudes, values and skills they need to keep themselves HIV free. It is precisely at this level that the greatest difficulties are encountered because many traditional curriculum approaches do not succeed in dealing appropriately with the issue of human sexuality or in bridging the communications gap with young people.

With some notable exceptions, the most commonly adopted curriculum perspective has been dominated by genitality – the particularised, physical consummation of the dynamic sexual energy that lies within each human being – and modes of HIV transmission. As a result, emphasis has tended to focus on biological and physiological issues, on risky behaviour, and on condom use. Some attention has been given to manifesting respect and regard for others in a spirit of equality and power-sharing that extends to all areas of life between males and females, but less to the meaning of sexuality, its role in relationships, and the norms for a joyful and healthy sexuality. Almost nothing suggests instruction about sexuality as a human drive for love, communion, community, friendship, family, self-perpetuation, happiness, humour and self-transcendence, or that the real good of human sexuality lies in contact with and surrender to the personality and not merely to the body of the partner.

From another perspective, having recognised the communications gap that can exist between them and younger people, an increasing number of educators are making room for peer education approaches that allow young people to have a say in what is presented and enable them to play an active role in interactive and participative presentations. This has been the cornerstone of the work of the Jamaica-based Ashe Ensemble in its work in Caribbean schools (*Box 6*). Others (so far very few) have gone beyond merely rational presentations, seeking, through Process Drama and other means, to establish emotional investment on the part of participants so that those involved take the message 'to heart', engage with it, reflect upon it, and ideally use it to shape their own conduct (Heap and Simpson, 2002).

Box 6.   The Ashe Edutainment Model

The Ashe edutainment methodology uses the performing arts to entertain, educate and empower audiences for behaviour transformation. Applying the Excitement, Involvement, Commitment (EIC) approach, the method shows participants how to be effective in adopting and passing on important messages. It excites through energisers, drama, music, dance and other performing arts; it involves participants in the creative process; thereby it empowers them to commit themselves to living, and teaching others to live, a lifestyle characterised by life-affirming choices.

Major goals of the activities are to:

- empower and transform young people to make positive choices and practice living a healthy lifestyle of abstinence, self-protection, and/or reclamation of their virginity;

- encourage young people to become involved in positive activities such as the performing arts or sports which will

Box 6 (cont'd).

keep them busy while they develop their talents, gifts and emotions;

• empower and transform parents, teachers and other adults to become knowledgeable and comfortable with their own sexuality so that they may feel free and confident to communicate with their children/students and guide them to live a healthy lifestyle;

• empower and transform parents, teachers and other adults to set positive examples for their young people to follow and live a healthy lifestyle.

These goals are achieved through performance and rap sessions that allow young people and their parents to 'get the facts' and learn the skills for managing their sexual world in an effective and non-preachy way. Through song, dance and drama, young people are helped in forming attitudes that will enable them to make positive life-affirming choices. A corresponding programme introduces parents to parenting tools, both positive (knowledge, communication, discipline and setting an example) and negative (ignorance, preaching, corporal punishment, mixed messages). The rap sessions allow for dialogue between the artistes and the audience in order to deepen the impact of the message and create an atmosphere where peer education can take place.

A manual is available for the training of teachers and guidance counsellors in using music and drama in behaviour development, specifically in the areas of sexuality development and HIV prevention (Robinson, 2002*a*). In addition, a second manual focuses on training parenting leaders (for example from PTAs) in the same areas to enable them to better communicate with their peers as parents and with their children (Robinson, 2002*b*).

These newer approaches are needed if messages about HIV/AIDS are to speak to young people, engage their interest and commitment, and promote real, personal assimilation of what has been learned or experienced. If education is really to be one of the world's most powerful forces against HIV/AIDS, then through these and other approaches the curriculum must enter into dialogue with the underlying cultural expressions which motivate young people from within, more powerfully than anything the educator may propose from without. Crucial aspects of these underlying cultural concerns include:

- the power of peer pressure and the group, and the need to conform and belong;

- the message implicitly learned from the failure of parents to discuss sex with their children, that sex is something which should not be discussed between adults and the young, but only between the young themselves, as equals;

- the socialization process which teaches boys that they must always and in all circumstances be 'physically strong, emotionally robust, daring and virile,' and that they should not depend on others, worry about their health, or seek help when they face problems (UNAIDS, 2000*a*);

- the widespread disbelief in the possibility of total sexual abstinence, particularly on the part of boys, and even some suspicion and concern that people who choose to abstain from sexual intercourse are abnormal or unhealthy. Accompanying this scepticism is a failure to provide the young with challenges and ideals that they will respect;

- the veneer of 'respectable', approved sexual behaviour encountered in society, while it is common knowledge that large numbers of adults are following a different sexual code;

- the double standards of societies that condone multiple partners for men and boys but condemn the same for women and girls;

- widespread and more-or-less accepted violence against women and girls;

- the way in which society condones or overlooks forced sex, at least so long as it does not extend beyond certain legally defined limits;

- the enormous mix of cultural values and counter-values coming from the weakening and progressive demise of traditional cultural systems, the importation of systems in which immediate pleasurable gratification becomes dominantly important, and the presentation by the entertainment industry of situations and role models which give prominence to temporary relationships and casual sex;

- the inadequate inculturation and socialization into respect for others as persons towards whom responsibility must be manifested and whose rights must be respected (UNECA, 2000:§48).

The education sector must also acknowledge that it has not been particularly successful in reaching young people including out-of-school children and youth outside the system. In some countries, the number of school-age children who are not in school exceeds the number who attend school. In the majority of countries, only a small minority of those in their late teens and twenties are in formal education programmes; the rest are either employed or are active in the non-formal sector in rural and urban areas, or would consider themselves as unemployed or idle. Responsibility for meeting the educational needs of this large cohort of young people usually rests with a variety of government ministries, depending on their sphere of responsibility. In practice, much of the thrust towards meeting the educational needs of young people who are not catered for by formal programmes rests with non-governmental, community and faith-based organizations.

The salience of young people for HIV/AIDS educational interventions cannot be overstated. If they can be saved from HIV infection and induced to provide care and support for those affected by the disease, the battle against AIDS will be won. But that battle is in danger of being lost because young people, those aged 15 to 24, constitute the highest risk age-group in the world, accounting for half the new infections each day. It is in relation to this group that the United Nations Declaration of Commitment has set for itself stringent targets:

- By 2003, establish time-bound national targets to achieve the internationally agreed global prevention goal to reduce by 2005 HIV prevalence among young men and women in the most affected countries by 25 per cent and by 25 per cent globally by 2010.

- By 2005, ensure that at least 90 per cent, and by 2010 at least 95 per cent of young men and women aged 15 to 24 have access to the information, education, including peer education and youthspecific HIV education, and services necessary to develop the life skills required to reduce their vulnerability to HIV infection (UNGASS, 2001:§47, 53).

Chapter 9 below considers information, education and communication strategies that have been adopted in Caribbean countries to bring HIV/ AIDS messages to young people outside the formal education system, and the potential for further multisectoral and multi-agency approaches in this area.

HIV/AIDS and the attainment of EFA goals

At the World Education Forum in Dakar in April 2000, the international community collectively committed itself to the attainment of six EFA goals relating to early childhood care and education, primary schooling for all, learning and life-skills programmes for all, more widespread adult literacy, the elimination of gender disparities in primary and secondary school systems, and improving all aspects of the quality of education. The forum further reaffirmed the need to implement as a matter of urgency education programmes and actions to combat the HIV/AIDS pandemic.

Ensuring progress towards the achievement of the EFA goals of primary schooling for all, the elimination of gender disparities in school systems, more universal adult literacy, and the improvement of all aspects of the quality of education, have long been the mainstay of educational development in many developing countries. Caribbean countries have dedicated themselves resolutely to the attainment of these goals. Although a great measure of success has attended their efforts, Caribbean personnel have identified a number of critical issues that still require attention in the region (*Box 7*).

Box 7. Critical issues identified in the Caribbean EFA 2000 reports

- Lack of access to primary education by marginalised groups in Caribbean societies.
- Early drop-out from basic education, particularly by males.
- Failure of the primary education system to produce high levels of literacy and numeracy.
- Weak systems for addressing post-school illiteracy among youths and adults.
- Increasing violence within educational institutions, particularly by teenage males against other students and their teachers.
- Lack of relevance of educational programming.
- Deterioration in teaching services and overall levels of professionalism, with inadequate preparation of teachers for programming requirements, falling status and esteem, and an exodus of teachers from the education systems of member states.

From the perspectives of both EFA goal attainment and HIV prevention education, the early drop-out from the basic education cycle, particularly by boys, is a matter of great concern. In many Caribbean countries the attendance and performance patterns in schools favour girls. Since the early 1990s, males have become more marginalised at all levels of the education system. Throughout the

English-speaking Caribbean, females are outstripping them in enrolment, attendance and performance. A major EFA challenge for the Caribbean education sector is to ensure that, in relation to young females, young males benefit equally from exposure to quality education.

The attainment of the EFA goals is closely intertwined with a successful response to HIV/AIDS. One cannot be realised without the other. In the words of the EFA Monitoring Report, 'There is increasing evidence that planning to achieve the EFA goals must take account of HIV/AIDS and that the spread and intensification of the pandemic will not be prevented in the absence of progress towards EFA' (UNESCO, 2002: 20). Because Caribbean males are not benefiting from EFA imperatives to the same extent as females, the potential impact of the HIV/AIDS epidemic on boys will require careful tracking across the region.

HIV/AIDS undercuts the ability to ensure more education, better education and gender-balanced education. As has been noted, in the most affected countries, children remain out of school; teachers become too few to meet the needs; teaching and learning are both impaired; resources are reduced; quality declines. But equally, more education, universal education, better education, and gender-balanced education, as envisaged at Dakar, undercut contextual and societal factors that would otherwise increase vulnerability to HIV infection. At the same time, well constructed and well delivered education has the potential to promote the positive attitudes and behaviours that avoid risk and manifest care and support.

By promoting the attainment of the EFA goals, education ministries are in fact making an effective response to the HIV/AIDS epidemic, even though they are not always expressly aware that they are doing so. Strategies and interventions developed at Cabinet, parliamentary and sectoral levels, as well as by regional and international aid agencies, should support them in this response, enabling its acceleration and scaling up. This is one sure way in which the education sector can make a significant contribution to the struggle with the epidemic.

CHAPTER 4

The Evolving Response of the Caribbean Education Sector to HIV/AIDS

The first two decades of the HIV/AIDS epidemic in the Caribbean saw the response largely concentrated within the health sector. HIV/ AIDS was regarded mostly as a health problem that required an appropriate health-based intervention. It is only in recent years that the wider social, cultural and economic implications of the epidemic have been recognised. In keeping with this approach, it is only in recent years that the need for an expanded response from the education sector has been considered.

During the first two decades of the epidemic, education's role tended to be concentrated in two areas – the provision of health education, including some HIV/AIDS-related education, to those attending school, and the strengthening of guidance and counselling within schools.

Confining education's response to HIV/AIDS to the fields of curriculum, guidance and counselling is not unique to the Caribbean. In the United States, the major thrust of the educational effort to deal with the epidemic is in the area of curriculum and school teaching programmes. This has been supported by the liberal commitment of extensive federal and state resources to school programmes dealing with reproductive health, abstinence, and ways of protecting oneself against HIV infection. The pattern of response has been much the same in other parts of the industrialised world. In a similar vein, investigations in Africa have revealed that up to the beginning of the twenty-first century the concern of the majority of education ministries was to incorporate HIV/AIDS into the curriculum and establish appropriate teaching programmes. They did not seem to be aware that they also had other responsibilities in relation to the epidemic, notably in the provision of care and support for infected and affected learners and educators, and in mitigating the negative impacts of the epidemic on the operations of the education system itself.

It is not surprising that education sectors across the world have responded in this way. Faced with an emerging problem, the dimensions of which were still unfolding, education sectors believed that since their comparative advantage lay in teaching they should adopt a teaching response to the epidemic. They were encouraged in this by popular views that expect school systems to provide the answers to problems affecting society, especially those affecting young people. Implicitly or explicitly school systems were challenged to 'do something about HIV/AIDS' by imparting knowledge and fostering attitudes and behaviours that would protect young people against HIV infection. Sometimes courageously, and sometimes timidly, persons within the education sector, including those in the Caribbean, took up this challenge. However, it would be fair to say that in many instances they did not always recognise the magnitude or scope of what they had undertaken. Neither did they recognise that they would have to incorporate into their plans and programmes many other dimensions if there was to be a comprehensive education response to HIV/AIDS.

Principal elements of the education sector's response to HIV/AIDS

In the 1980s and 1990s international understanding of the potential of the education sector to contribute to the containment of the AIDS epidemic was quite limited, while the appreciation of the potential of the epidemic to undermine the education sector was almost non-existent. Given this context, it should come as no surprise that responses to a survey conducted in 1999 on curriculum development needs at the upper primary and secondary education levels in the Caribbean made no reference to HIV/AIDS (IBE, 1999). Although the questionnaire dealt with priority areas of concern in curriculum content and priority needs for regional cooperation, the respondents made no mention of HIV/AIDS. Clearly, the need for the education sector to play a role in HIV prevention and in mitigating the impacts of the epidemic in the region had not yet been fully appreciated. At that time, and for several years previously, the HIV response of the education sector was focused in two broad areas:

1.   Establishing links between school health and education, the principal concern being with the Health and Family Life Education (HFLE) initiative; and

2.   Strengthening guidance and counselling (in some countries).

In addition, some knowledge, attitude, behaviour and practice (KABP) studies were undertaken in a few countries. These were of considerable value in the way they extended knowledge and understanding of behavioural responses to the epidemic. They tended, however, to be country specific and did not form part of any comprehensive investigation across the region.

Development of the health and family life education initiative

The HFLE initiative[1] in the Caribbean has had a relatively long developmental history. The programme was commissioned in response to the desire of Caribbean governments to equip the region's youth to cope better with the situations that arise from changing societal and family values and traditions, the perception of disintegrating community life, and the development of new health problems. The initiative is a CARICOM multi-agency activity that seeks to empower young people with skills for healthy living and focuses on the development on the whole person (emotional, social, mental, physical and spiritual). The programme is implemented through a partnership arrangement between the CARICOM Secretariat, various UN agencies, the University of the West Indies (UWI), expert consultants on HFLE, and the education and health ministries of fourteen CARICOM countries.

HIV/AIDS was not the principal impetus for introducing this comprehensive approach. Although the epidemic was looming as a major regional issue in the early 1990s, a more dominant role in triggering the HFLE initiative was regional concern over a variety of health and social problems in such areas as adolescent pregnancy, violence, family breakdown, substance abuse, and obesity. In a number of countries the initiative was initially spearheaded by the Ministry of Health, but subsequently was gradually transferred to education ministries. Thus, in the Eastern Caribbean the HFLE programme currently pertains to the ministries responsible for education, youth, and health while in Jamaica it is located in the guidance and counselling division of the Ministry of Education.

In the first half of the 1990s, the HFLE initiative targeted policymakers in the health and education sectors with a view of bringing existing programmes into line with the more comprehensive HFLE approach and to having the subject area adopted as a core subject in the school curriculum. Activities continued throughout the 1990s to strengthen HFLE in the formal and non-formal education sectors. Despite the decision by the Ministers of Education in 1996 that HFLE be treated as a core subject in the school curriculum, with status equivalent to that of English or mathematics, the consensus is that insufficient progress has been made in its implementation in the schools.

At first the programme was introduced in some secondary schools, with a gradual extension to primary schools (and in several cases totally absent). However, the full integration of the programme into the school curriculum has been slowed down by three factors that are still being addressed: the training of HFLE facilitators and teachers, the development of HFLE curriculum outlines for pre-primary, primary and secondary schools, and the development and production of classroom materials to support the teaching of HFLE in schools.

An early decision to have HFLE included as a core subject for certification in teacher training colleges in the Eastern Caribbean still awaits implementation, although agreement has been reached that teachers' colleges throughout the region include a minimum level of instruction in HFLE areas for all trainees. But this agreement still needs to be widened to ensure that those graduating from teacher training institutions are adequately equipped to deliver HIV/AIDS education programmes in the classroom.

With technical guidance from the Pan-American Health Organization (PAHO) some progress has been made in the preparation of new core HFLE curriculum guidelines for pre-primary, primary and secondary schools. The process of defining the key elements and approaches for curriculum development for CARICOM schools has been initiated, but guidelines for the core curriculum areas have yet to be made available to relevant personnel across the region.

Concerning HIV/AIDS, the situation in regard to classroom materials remains even more critical. While there are some materials that support the general HFLE programme, a survey in 2002 found that apart from one academic reader there were no books on HIV/AIDS for the Commonwealth Caribbean, and no books or workbooks on the subject for general use in schools (Morrissey, 2002). Findings from the survey pointed to the need for school materials to be published in the context of national policy and with support from national education ministries, in cooperation with faith-based organisations, school boards, AIDS organisations, and others. In the absence of such approved materials, even teachers who are positively disposed to teaching about HIV/AIDS will not be able to do so.

Policy development, with regard to both the HFLE initiative and HIV/AIDS imperatives, is making slow headway. In 1996 education ministers requested all CARICOM states to develop national HFLE policies and prepare plans of action for the translation of that policy into action, but at the time of writing only five countries had approved HFLE policies. With regard to HIV/AIDS, apart from Haiti (below), no country has articulated a comprehensive, fully developed policy to guide the education sector's response. Some elements may be in place, relating for instance to dealing with the epidemic in schools or the workplace, but throughout the Commonwealth Caribbean and beyond, the sector still awaits the development of an HIV/AIDS-in-education policy framework that takes account of all the complexities and implications of the epidemic.

Guidance and counselling

Other than in Haiti, no education ministry in the region has signalled its intention of creating a dedicated structure that would have the sole function of dealing with HIV/AIDS in the sector. Instead the approach has been to entrust responsibility for HIV/AIDS to existing sub-units or divisions. The task of responding to the epidemic and of mitigating its impacts has been added to the workload of these units (and in territories with small populations, to the workload of individual officers). Understandably, these units and officers tend to interpret the epidemic and its impacts in terms of their current areas of specialization. Many of them are also aware that their understanding of HIV/AIDS and the way it can impact the education sector is not very extensive. They experience a genuine need to develop their capacity to guide the education sector's response to the epidemic.

Because HIV prevention is most often viewed in terms of behaviour change, a number of ministries took the logical step of entrusting responsibility for HIV/AIDS issues to their guidance and counselling units or divisions. Starting from the time when the epidemic began to be taken on board by education ministries, these have been the principal units within the sector active in the HIV/AIDS arena. Their accomplishments have included the promotion of safe behaviour messages through the HFLE curriculum, capacity building at school level through the training of teachers and guidance counsellors in relevant skills, extensive awareness raising and sensitisation activities, and the establishment of community networks representative of parents, community organisations and the general public. However, in terms of national needs, the coverage of these programmes has been far from complete.

Given that the AIDS epidemic continues to grow in the region and that the prospects are that it will be several years before it finally peaks, education ministries will need to reconsider the practice of extending the workload of a unit or individual by simply adding on responsibility for HIV/AIDS in the sector. The AIDS situation is of such gravity, and the implications for sector activity are so complex, that ministries in larger territories may need to consider establishing dedicated units to manage the problem. In territories with small populations, the need may be to relieve an individual of some part of other responsibilities to allow for greater concentration of effort on the problems raised by HIV/AIDS in the sector.

Overview of HIV/AIDS-and-education sector interventions in the Caribbean

In keeping with the understanding that, first and foremost, HIV/AIDS was a health problem, the major thrust of support to the Caribbean education sector in the area of HIV/AIDS has been from a health perspective. Initiatives supported or developed by regional and United Nations agencies (CARICOM, CAREC, UNESCO, UNICEF, UNDP, UNIFEM, UNFPA, PAHO/WHO) dealt predominantly with school health activities and principally with developing the HFLE programme. Apart from the HFLE, some other current programmes are also oriented strongly towards the health domain – for instance, the Caribbean Network for Health Promoting Schools, established in 1998. In general terms, the thrust of efforts in the 1990s was mostly towards curriculum development for school health programmes and some strengthening of teacher training to be able to implement new health-related curriculum initiatives. HIV/AIDS fell within these parameters and did not usually receive specific attention as a separate issue.

There were, however, exceptions. As early as 1996, Barbados conducted an evaluation in several schools and developed a comprehensive HIV/AIDS programme for primary education. Beginning in 1997, the 'Life After School' project was initiated in several Eastern Caribbean and other countries; the project targets high school students in their final years to increase their knowledge about HIV/AIDS and orient them towards a productive AIDS-free life. Since 1998 Haiti has been implementing on an ever more extensive basis its 'Education to Family Life' programme that deals with knowledge, attitudes and values relating to reproductive health and population.

Since about 2000, some changes have occurred in the type of HIV/AIDS intervention being made in the Caribbean education sector.

Health continues to be the principal perspective, but there are now more programmes that focus specifically on HIV/AIDS or deal with issues that arise from the epidemic. For instance, Barbados has conducted a knowledge, attitudes, beliefs and practices (KABP) study to asses the knowledge, attitudes, and values of young people in relation to HIV/AIDS and the gender and human rights dimensions of the epidemic (*Box 8*). Barbados and Jamaica have both developed HIV/AIDS resource materials for those with learning difficulties or special needs. Guyana has established a 'Youth Challenge and HIV/ AIDS' programme that seeks to increase the level of information and knowledge on HIV/AIDS among 12 to 15 year-old youth through music, dance and the arts. The project, 'A Force to Reckon: Youth Against AIDS in the Caribbean', which is being piloted in Barbados prior to eventual extension throughout the region, seeks to empower youth and educate them to advocate for human rights in the face of widespread HIV/AIDS-related stigma and discrimination. In Jamaica, the 'Youth at the Crossroads' programmes target some adolescents, in and out of school, for HIV/AIDS prevention and life skills development.

Box 8. Conclusions of the Barbados KABP Study

'This exploratory study revealed high levels of knowledge and relatively positive attitudes and beliefs. Nevertheless, there were several inconsistencies across and within the areas under investigation and a number of issues that emerged as a cause for concern. Although the respondents (more than 90.0%) displayed familiarity with, and significant knowledge of, most modes of transmission, ignorance of some basic facts of transmissibility continues to exist. Other instances of inconsistency were revealed between

- knowledge and attitudes and beliefs;

Box 8 (cont'd).

- knowledge and sexual practices; and
- attitudes and beliefs and sexual practices.

The survey shows that considerable education in relation to HIV/AIDS remains to be done among young people regarding body fluids such as saliva and urine as well as medical procedures such as giving blood and having a blood test.

In respect of sexual practice, the triad of early onset of sexual intercourse, multiple partners and inconsistent condom use remain major challenges in dealing with the disease. In similar vein, there is evidence that the socio-cultural context of sexual activity frequently compounds the problem as substantial proportions of respondents indicated having had sex when drunk or high, or having had sex without a condom because their partner did not want to use one....

The fact that the majority of respondents did not find the current HIV/AIDS programmes to be effective is a sobering finding....

The survey confirms that whereas education and sensitisation remain important responses to the HIV/AIDS epidemic, the more difficult and urgent challenge is translating knowledge and information into appropriate behaviour. There is an insistent call from respondents in this survey for changes in the methodologies and approaches to public sensitisation. There is a call to put a human face on the epidemic and to move the public education out of the sterile, abstract world of statistics and factual statements.'

Source: Ministry of Education, Youth and Sport, Barbados, 2001: 40-41.

In addition, various youth education and empowerment programmes (including the continuation of the 'Life after School' initiative) have been established in Antigua, the British Virgin Islands, Grenada, Montserrat, St. Lucia, St. Vincent and the Grenadines, and Suriname. Many of these programmes rely heavily on a peer education approach and make extensive use of the media. Some of the programmes are conducted in schools, both primary and secondary, while some seek alternative ways of reaching young people. The focus of all of them is quite expressly HIV/AIDS, its implications, how to prevent its transmission, how to relate to those who are infected or affected, and how to manage some of the negative impacts of the epidemic.

A continuing issue of concern with these and other programmes is that so many of them remain small-scale. There is a great deal of focus on pilot projects and experimental activities, but much less attention to taking any of them to scale. An additional concern is the absence of textbooks, readers, and other resource materials that have been formally approved for use in schools and are made available through the normal official education system channels. Almost all of the materials that have been developed have originated with non-governmental or faith-based organizations (NGOs/FBOs). In terms of content, some of these seem to merit wider dissemination. But this is an undertaking that belongs more properly to education ministries than to NGOs or FBOs. The development and dissemination of a sustainable supply of quality school learning materials for HIV/AIDS and related areas are major priorities for education ministries in the region.

It is clear from this overview that HIV/AIDS interventions in the Caribbean education sector:

- still focus strongly on school health programmes;
- except for the HFLE multi-agency initiative, tend to be individual, uncoordinated projects of relatively short duration;
- have become much more explicitly concerned in recent years with HIV/AIDS and its implications for personal living;
- are not yet supported by the necessary resource materials;

- have been directed mostly towards HIV prevention among young people, but have not been concerned with the impacts of the epidemic on the education sector.

In respect of the last point, the Caribbean Ministers of Education have acknowledged the potential of HIV/AIDS to deplete the human resources needed for sustainable development in the Caribbean and, in their Havana Commitment (frontispiece), have recognised the importance of creative measures to reduce the impact of the epidemic on the education sector. The Ministers' concern is being followed up by an ongoing joint UNESCO-CARICOM initiative to develop a major programme that will strengthen the capacity of the education sector of every country in the region to maximize its contribution to HIV/ AIDS prevention and to mitigate the effects of the epidemic on its operations. Integral to this development will be situation and response analyses that, among other things, will assess the direct and indirect impacts of HIV/AIDS on the education sector.

Haiti's strategic plan for education and HIV/AIDS

Haiti is experiencing a very severe HIV/AIDS epidemic. Estimates are that the prevalence rate in the 15 to 49 year-old age group is 6.1 per cent; that there are between 240,000 and 335,000 persons in the country living with the disease; and that 25 to 40 thousand new cases of HIV infection occur each year. In response to these realities and recognising its responsibility to protect the human capital of the nation, especially in children and the youth, the Ministry of Education, Youth and Sport (MENJS) undertook the development of a strategic plan that would draw maximum benefit from education in the struggle against HIV/AIDS (Haiti, 2002). This is the first national strategic plan for HIV/AIDS and Education in the Caribbean and still one of the very few in the world. As such it deserves special consideration and, where appropriate, emulation.

The plan comprises three parts:

1. An HIV/AIDS situation analysis, from the perspective of the economy, socio-cultural features, and national HIV/AIDS plans

on the one hand; and from the perspective of educational provision, accomplishments, constraints, and opportunities on the other.

2. The broad outlines of how the education sector proposes to respond to the epidemic.

3. Implementation and action strategies, with special reference to the structural arrangements required to initiate and maintain action.

The education ministry in Haiti believes that, in the circumstances of the epidemic, its primary responsibilities are to contribute to HIV prevention and to reduce the impact of the disease on the education community. The guiding principles that governed the development of the plan were based on considerations of ethics, values and human rights. These served to embed the plan firmly in a human rights based framework. They consisted of six principles:

1. Recognition that the struggle against HIV/AIDS is a priority for the education ministry.

2. An approach to HIV/AIDS anchored firmly in human rights considerations.

3. The need to break the silence and speak openly about HIV/AIDS, while at the same time eliminating such negative features as stigma, discrimination, sexual violence, and sexual abuse.

4. The protection of human capital as the key to future development.

5. The need to ensure a secure learning environment in respect to the health and HIV/AIDS needs of every member of the education community.

6. The need to ensure coordination on the part of all stakeholders and partners.

In the light of the education ministry's vision and guiding principles, the plan outlines the strategic choices that will guide it in its work of responding to HIV/AIDS:

1. Ensure that all young people, especially those in difficult circumstances, have access to basic education for a sufficient

number of years. Among other things, this strategy highlights the importance of ensuring that girls have equal access to education.

2. Develop the necessary policies and codes of procedure, particularly those needed to ensure a safe school environment and zero tolerance for sexual abuse, sexual harassment, and all other forms of school-related violence.

3. Reinforce and develop at all levels – from pre-school to university – health and HIV/AIDS education programmes.

4. By the provision of adequate teaching space, teaching materials, hygienic conditions, and basic health and psycho-social services, establish a supportive environment for the learning process and learning activities.

5. Strengthen and develop programmes for children and youth in difficult situations, such as orphans, street children, migrants, handicapped children, or children in domestic service.

6. Integrate the community fully into all education activities and specifically into HIV prevention programmes. This strategy calls for greater alignment between the education provided by the school and that given in the home.

7. Develop a communications programme that, among other things, will capitalize on the potential of both traditional and technological media. This strategy also underlines the importance of ensuring consensus and the absence of conflict in the messages that all parties communicate to the young.

8. Establish a monitoring and evaluation system that will generate information on health and HIV/AIDS in the education sector.

9. Develop a wide range of partnerships and foster a multi-sectoral approach, in order to ensure better coordination, wider access to resources, clarification of roles and responsibilities, and better geographical coverage.

Finally, in terms of structure, the plan proposes the establishment of a high-level inter-sectoral committee, chaired by the Minister of

Education, Youth and Sport, to serve as a consultative board that will give guidance in the entire area of HIV/AIDS in education. At the operational level, it provides for an HIV/AIDS coordinating unit directly responsible to the ministry's Director-General and working with its technical directorates (for pre-school, basic, secondary, and higher education, and for scientific research) and partners to direct the implementation of the plan.

In many respects, Haiti's development of its strategic plan for HIV/AIDS and the education sector marks the culmination of a process that is still at an early stage in other countries. In some it has not even been started. A major strength of Haiti's initiative is the prominence given from the outset to ethical values, and human rights considerations. Apart from HIV/AIDS concerns, these inter-related issues should be prominent in all planning for the development and consolidation of the education sector. They provide the rationale for the millennium development goals that the world is striving to achieve. They also underpin the global approach to responding to HIV/AIDS, as expressed by the United Nations in its Declaration of Commitment on HIV/AIDS when it recognized that 'the full realization of human rights and fundamental freedoms for all is an essential element in a global response to the HIV/AIDS pandemic' (UNGASS, 2001:§16). In this and other respects Haiti has marked out a path that, with modifications to suit their circumstances, other countries could well follow.

Note

1. This section deals with the development of this programme and the action of education ministries. The programme content and objectives are dealt with in *Chapter 6*.

ADDRESSING THE EPIDEMIC

CHAPTER 5

New Roles for Education

After almost two decades of uncertainty, the world has come to acknowledge that HIV/AIDS is more than a health issue. It now recognises with increasing clarity that it is a development issue that reaches into every area of human endeavour. Likewise, in the field of education, the epidemic is not something that the sector can address merely by incorporating HIV/AIDS, sexual and reproductive health and life-skills into teaching programmes. There are numerous other aspects to the challenge posed by the disease that must be given their due weight in educational programmes and institutions. Important perspectives relate to such areas as:

- Counteracting denial, fear and discrimination.
- Ensuring access to the necessary psycho-social counselling for pupils, teachers and administrators.
- Ensuring care and support for infected and affected learners and educators.
- Promoting an institutional environment that is safe and supportive.
- Protecting every employee, whether working in a school or elsewhere within the education system, from HIV infection.
- Extending and strengthening links between schools and communities.

Counteracting denial, fear and discrimination

As a medical condition, HIV/AIDS is probably unique in the way it is wrapped in layer upon layer of denial, fear, and discrimination. It is commonly found that individuals and communities experience a strong inclination to maintain silence about certain personal or family medical problems, such as cancer, epilepsy or mental illness. But these and similar conditions are not cloaked with denial, secrecy, fear, stigma, prejudice and discrimination to the same extent as HIV/ AIDS.

Stigma, silence and perpetuation of the spread of HIV are intimately connected. 'Stigma remains our most significant challenge in responding to HIV/AIDS. It makes prevention through education very difficult. Eliminating it must be central in the response to AIDS. It is a key way to break the silence and move the response forward' (Peter Piot, Address at Opening Ceremony, Eleventh ICASA Conference, Lusaka, 12 September, 1999). 'The fear of stigma leads to silence, and when it comes to fighting AIDS, silence is death. It suppresses public discussion about AIDS, and deters people from finding out whether they are infected' (Kofi Annan, Message for World AIDS Day 2002).

Denial occurs when an individual, institution, sector or country does not face up to the relevance of HIV/AIDS to their circumstances. This may occur because they want to shut themselves off from a reality that is too hard to bear. More often, however, they do not want to admit that a disease that spreads mostly by behaviour labelled as 'immoral' could cause a problem within their families, communities or country (UNAIDS, 2000b: 38). Fear arises from the instinctual perception that the basic channels of human life and continuity – blood, sexual intercourse, giving birth, mother's milk – are now potential channels of sickness and death. The fear is aggravated by the mistaken view that AIDS is rapidly and inevitably fatal, and is compounded by the many misconceptions that HIV can be contracted from casual or social interaction with an infected person, almost as if it were a contagious disease transmitted through the air or by non-sexual touch.

With such origins, denial and fear readily lead to stigma. Stigma is very close to negative prejudice. Both imply judging adversely the worth and dignity of another on insufficient or irrelevant grounds, such as race, colour, religion, language, or HIV/AIDS status. Individuals who hold such prejudiced viewpoints or positions may take actions that negatively impact on the rights and entitlements of others. If they do so, they act out their stigma and thereby discriminate against others. In this way, stigma and discrimination are closely linked. But even in the absence of active discriminatory action, stigma has other negative consequences. The individual who is stigmatised will almost always recognise the prejudice that underlies the way she or he is regarded. This damages the sense of acceptance and approval that is vital to much of human interaction, and, in the case of HIV, leads to great reluctance on the part of infected or affected individuals and families to reveal their status, lest they experience scorn, disdain, or hostility on the part of others. Infected and affected persons also tend to experience a diminished sense of self-worth and self-esteem and heightened feelings of guilt and self-blame. This is because they think that their HIV status or even their proximity to the disease makes them feared, abhorred, blamed, or regarded as 'different'. In all too many cases, their experience bears out the truth of this thinking.

As in so many other parts of the world, HIV/AIDS in the Caribbean is coupled with an extensive reaction of fear and prejudice (*Box 9*). There is also a large admixture of ignorance. In many instances these factors have resulted in 'marginalisation, stigma and outright discrimination and violation of the human rights of people infected and living with HIV/AIDS' (CRSPAH), 2000: 10).

Box 9. HIV-positive in Trinidad and in fear of discrimination

I am 22 years old. I found out I am positive after I went to an STD clinic with my boyfriend, who tested positive for another STD. Then I found out I had HIV. I live with my mother and grandmother and if they found out about me [being HIV positive] they would put me out of the house. They are not educated enough to accept me if that information is shared. They would be scared and feel they would get it from casual contact. If my boss found out, I know he would definitely fire me (Voisin and Dillon-Remy, 2001: 79).

The education sector has a multiple role in responding to this situation. First, education ministries need to establish a clear regulatory framework. This should be solidly rights based but at the same time should give guidance on practical ways of minimizing the risks of HIV transmission. It would be preferable that, in developing such a code of procedure, education ministries work in partnership with teacher unions, parent representatives and leaders of faith-based organisations. Moreover, given that stigma and discrimination are so widespread in the Caribbean, it would be desirable to develop a user-friendly version of such a manual for use by school boards and parent-teacher committees. This would help to ensure the concerted action of the entire school community in counteracting HIV/AIDS-related denial, fear and discrimination.

Second, ministries must robustly ensure that every educational institution and setting manifests a welcoming approach for infected and affected individuals and zero tolerance for any discriminatory action. School principals and teachers need to be helped to recognise that even though the sickness of HIV or AIDS may affect only a few, the malady of stigma and discrimination is much more widespread and is something that every educational institution must seek to remedy. School authorities need to be particularly on the alert to ensure the complete absence of the petty taunting and mockery that pupils indulge in so easily and that can bring untold misery to a fellow-learner who is already striving to cope with HIV/AIDS at home or somewhere within the family circle. Even where there may be no overt discrimination against them, infected or affected learners or educators may experience subtle forms of prejudice and ostracism.

The third area where the education sector can take action is by school authorities taking steps to ensure that every pupil has sufficient knowledge of HIV/AIDS to dispel commonly held fears and prejudices, and recognises that there are no grounds for stigmatizing any infected or affected person, whether in the school or elsewhere. The attitude they should strive to promote is that 'my friend with AIDS is still my friend'. Some of this work will have to be done in the classroom, using whatever opportunities present themselves to deal with HIV/AIDS from a human rights perspective. Data from the Barbados KABP survey showed that although the majority of respondents were generally sympathetic to HIV persons, there remained a small proportion that advocated isolation, thereby demonstrating a mixture of fear, ignorance and intolerance. The report noted that 'such attitudes would need to be addressed through a comprehensive programme of education and counselling' (Barbados, 2001: 21). If it is to provide such a comprehensive programme, the HFLE curriculum may need extension and strengthening so that it could include a component on ethics, values and human rights, with special attention to stigma and discrimination.

Recognising that violence, substance abuse and disregard for the environment constitute further major problems in the region, any HFLE revision should also make room for curriculum attention to the values and human rights implications of these areas. Moreover, in addition to classroom activity, opportunities arise for education across this whole domain of values, attitudes and human rights in school assemblies and, with the cooperation of the religious authorities, on the occasions when the school meets for worship. What is important is that sensitivity to the human rights of every person becomes a core value in every school, permeating the school culture and manifesting itself in zero tolerance for stigma and discrimination towards those infected or affected by HIV/AIDS.

Counselling

Apart from the stigma and discrimination so frequently associated with it, HIV/AIDS gives rise to considerable trauma and psychological distress, especially among the young. Educators and school heads may be at a loss as to how they should cope with this. In particular they need to be better supported in assisting learners from families where there is HIV or AIDS and in responding to the ensuing range of emotional, psychological and behavioural problems that these may present. Experience from other parts of the world shows that because of HIV/AIDS, schools are increasingly becoming home to growing numbers of learners who are dysfunctional intellectually, socially and psychologically, but little provision is made to enable school authorities deal with these disadvantaged young people. A special challenge that many schools experience is in responding appropriately to the psycho-social problems experienced by orphans. In addition, the epidemic is also causing emotional and psychological distress for teachers and administrators themselves.

These considerations point to the fact that HIV/AIDS has accentuated the need for a cadre of well-trained guidance and counselling personnel who can respond to the requirements of both learners and educators in schools. This need in relation to HIV/AIDS is in line with another requirement identified in many parts of the Caribbean, namely the need to strengthen preventive mental health services for children, adolescents and young adults in view of the high levels of stress being experienced by today's youth and the special challenges presented by issues such as violence and drug abuse. What Williams says of Jamaica may well be applicable to territories elsewhere in the region: 'There is an urgent need for adolescents to have access to counselling services to deal with the emotional and psychological trauma caused by exposure to violence' (Williams, 2002: 269).

Clearly, the role of counsellors in school life must be reviewed. Education sector leaders are responsible for ensuring that this is done. As a recommended first step, authorities in several Caribbean countries might take action to increase the pool of trained guidance counsellors and to ensure that these persons can provide their professional services to students and teachers in primary and secondary schools.

Expanding the cadre of counselling personnel will require enlarged and possibly revamped programmes in universities and training institutions. Recognising the extent of this challenge, teacher training colleges and other tertiary level institutions may need to take action along two dimensions:

- incorporating aspects of guidance and counselling more comprehensively in all teacher preparation programmes, so that every teacher is equipped with some of the basics in this area; and

- reversing the low priority given to specialist certificate, diploma and degree programmes in guidance and counselling.

In this context, positive moves have been the launching of a new degree programme in guidance and counselling at Mico Teachers' College in Jamaica, the proposal for a new UWI certificate programme for the training of HIV/AIDS counsellors and prevention assistants, and the strengthening of existing programmes in counselling and counselling psychology at theological colleges. The UWI initiative has the added value of including special provision for the participation of HIV-positive trainees in the programme, a move that gives reason to believe that the new programme will be firmly rooted in the realities and needs of those who experience the psycho-social turmoil that HIV/AIDS can occasion.

Care and support for infected and affected learners and educators

Where the AIDS epidemic is generalised, reaching beyond high risk groups into the general population, it can be expected that a certain proportion of children of school age, as well as a number of teachers and other education staff, will be HIV infected. Some of the children may have received the infection from their mothers during pregnancy or delivery or when breast-feeding. Child abuse and exploitation, which appear to be as widespread in the Caribbean as in other countries, may be responsible for the infection of some. Still others may have become infected through sexual activity, especially since the pattern of early sexual initiation, common in Caribbean countries, usually brings with it a high risk of HIV infection. The PAHO adolescent survey (*Figure 2*) provides clear regional evidence on the very early age at which sexual activity commences for both boys and girls. Becoming sexually active at a very early age increases the risk of HIV infection, especially for girls, and hence accentuates the possibility of HIV infected students being enrolled in the upper classes of primary school and at all levels in secondary school.

Notwithstanding their generally higher level of education, teachers and other education staff in countries with a generalised epidemic may experience the same risk of HIV infection as others in the community. Even though education and understanding of the disease offer some protection against the risk of infection, it does not follow that educators always allow the logic of that education to work its way out in their own personal lives. For educators, decisions about HIV prevention may pay more regard to powerful emotional feelings than to rational, volitional thinking.

The possibility that HIV may be present in an educational institution, and that in the case of older personnel it may progress to AIDS, underscores the need for every institution to be ready to cope with HIV/AIDS as a feature of its day-to-day institutional life. In a world with HIV/AIDS, every institution, including every school, must be prepared to ensure an environment of care and support for those who are infected, once their HIV status is known. *Box 10* itemises several initiatives that education managers can take.

Box 10. Care and support initiatives for infected learners and educators

1. Establish an atmosphere of acceptance and welcome where there will be no suspicion, no anxiety on anybody's part, no patronizing of those who are infected, and a complete absence of stigma and discrimination.

2. Establish a climate of normality that does not single out the individual living with HIV/AIDS for any special treatment or consideration, but accepts the occurrence of the disease in much the same way that it accepts other medical conditions. This involves making it clear to all concerned that, unless medically indicated, students or staff living with HIV/AIDS will be treated no differently from others in their group. In particular, all should be clear that, in the absence of other supportive medical evidence, HIV infection alone will not be taken as sufficient reason for failing to perform work, complete assignments, attend classes, or write/mark examinations.

3. Make special provisions to enable those whose work is interrupted by illness to make up for lost time and catch up on lost opportunities. Responding to this need in a student or teacher can be a very practical expression of acceptance.

4. Where the situation warrants it, make flexible provisions that will support home-based study or work on the part of an infected learner or educator. This flexibility could extend also to the way the school day is arranged, taking into account the pressures female staff or girls may experience if they are caring for an AIDS patient in their homes. It could also extend to financial requirements, in view of the tendency for AIDS-affected households to have to increase their outlays while experiencing reduced incomes.

5. Having ascertained that this is what the parents or guardians of infected learners, or infected educators themselves, would want, establish systems that would allow social, welfare and medical providers to intervene when infected individuals need their services. It would be valuable to explore the possibility of involving the wider community of parents, and of community

Box 10 (cont'd).

and faith-based organisations, in aspects of these services, such as in providing transport or nutritious meals.

6. Arrange for those who are infected to have ready access to qualified counsellors.

7. In collaboration with parents, community and faith-based organisations, provide for the financial, social and interactive personal support that will enable learners or educators who have HIV or AIDS to live in human dignity, peace and hope.

8. Wherever it seems appropriate, encourage students or educators living with HIV/AIDS to divulge their status, and enhance their sense of self-worth by enabling them to play a strong leadership and advocacy role in the institution's struggle with HIV/AIDS.

9. Ensure that as part of their general education everybody in the school is well acquainted with the ways that HIV can and cannot be transmitted. While it would be advisable to post universal precautions (*Box 11*) on bulletin boards in staff rooms, laboratories and other key places, it is also important that the risks of accidental HIV infection through contact with the blood of infected learners or educators should not be exaggerated.

10. Promote the availability and use of voluntary counselling and testing services. Among other things, access to such services would help to defuse potential hysteria situations that might arise among school students who learn that one of their colleagues is HIV positive and fear it may be the same for themselves.

11. Ensure that action is taken on the basic components of the FRESH initiative (*Chapter 6* – health-related school policies, provision of safe water and adequate sanitation, skills-based health education, and school-based health and nutrition services.

These are areas in which schools have not traditionally been involved. But they are areas that, in the circumstances of HIV/AIDS, school managers, governing bodies and parent associations cannot ignore. The positive side of intervention along the lines proposed is the way they would help to bind a school together as a community.

They would also help to strengthen the school's relations with the community it serves, thereby narrowing a gap that the school's concentration on its strictly academic functions tends to maintain.

Box 11. Universal or standard precautions

'Universal precautions' are simple standards of infection control practices to be used in interacting with persons who are HIV positive to minimise the risk of blood-borne pathogens. They are called universal precautions because it is recommended that they be applied to all persons, regardless of what their HIV status might be. Universal precautions consist of:

- Careful handling and disposal of sharp objects (needles, razors, or other objects with a sharp point or edge).

- Hand-washing before and after a procedure.

- Using protective barriers – such as gloves, masks, gowns – when there is direct contact with blood or other body fluids. Where gloves are not available, intact plastic bags that do not have holes can provide the necessary protection for the hands.

- Disposing in a safe way waste items that have been in direct contact with blood or other body fluids.

- Disinfecting in a proper way instruments and other equipment that may have been in direct contact with blood or other body fluids.

- Handling linen or garments that may have been in direct contact with blood or other body fluids in a proper way (avoiding direct contact with the soiled area, wearing gloves, etc.).

Source: Edited from *An ILO Code of Practice on HIV/AIDS and the World of Work*, International Labour Office, Geneva, 2001: 23.

Make the school environment safe and supportive

Every society is confronted by a need to deal with violence and reduce its extent and negative consequences, and the Caribbean is no different. In parts of the region, however, issues of violence have become so embedded in public awareness that some experts regard reducing the level of violence as the most dominant social concern facing the Caribbean. In the immediate, vehement and destructive way that it impinges on community life in many territories, violence seems to dwarf HIV/AIDS in the public consciousness. Yet the two are linked, especially for young people. The situation of violence creates conditions that facilitate HIV transmission, as instanced by rape, child abuse, drug trafficking, and the disintegration of the social norms that in an earlier period reduced the likelihood of risky sexual behaviour. Clearly, the way young girls are forced to endure 'the hidden story of coercive sex, rape, incest, (and) domestic violence' (CRSPAH, 2000: 9) accentuates the risk that they will become HIV infected. On the other hand, HIV can give rise to violence, for example, when allegations that an individual or family member is HIV-positive lead to verbal, emotional and physical aggression.

Schools are not exempt from this atmosphere of violence. In some extreme cases, students may be afraid to go to school because of ongoing violence in the community or on the streets but remain at home until the violence cools off (UNESCO/UNFPA, 2002: 27). In other cases they fear being accosted and possibly abused on the way to or from school. Within the school itself, violence also manifests itself, between students themselves and between students and teachers (*Box 7*). To some extent violence is even institutionalised in practices of corporal punishment and maintaining control through beatings, angry verbal confrontations, and other forms of aggression. While these are not as prominent as in the past, the traditions have not entirely died away. An investigation in one country in 2001 found that almost all the teachers surveyed used corporal punishment, and likewise almost all of the children reported that they had received corporal punishment, mostly in the form of being slapped, but also in other forms, such as being made to stand in the sun or to kneel (Meeks Gardner *et al.*, 2001, in Williams, 2002).

A further aspect of school violence that is more immediately relevant to HIV/AIDS is the extent to which school-related sexual activity takes place. Many countries across the world are unearthing distressing evidence of school children being abused by teachers in return for the payment of school fees, the promise of good examination grades, appointment to positions of responsibility and leadership, or for the sheer gratification of teacher power. Evidence also continues to emerge of younger children, boys as well as girls, being abused by older pupils. Systematic evidence about the extent to which these offences occur in Caribbean schools is sparse, but on the basis of what has become known about other societies the possibility of such transgressions must be allowed for. This area, and the related area of the protection of the rights of the child in school settings, merit further investigation in Caribbean countries.

A primary response to these interlocking problems is to ensure that schools provide a safe and supportive environment for young people. From the management aspect, this means zero tolerance for acts of sexual violence, harassment or exploitation against children and adolescents, and particularly against girls. School authorities, governing bodies, and parent associations must take every necessary step to make school-related sexual violence completely unacceptable, and they need to be backed up in their endeavours by clear policies established and enforced by education ministries.

From the education perspective, the life-skills component of the HFLE curriculum provides schools with scope to extend their treatment of conflict resolution to cover ways of dealing constructively with the conflict and violence situations that arise in all areas of life, in addition to strengthening capacity to resolve conflicts in areas of sexual practice or activity. A more express school focus on learning to live together, one of the four pillars of learning proposed by UNESCO (1996: 85-95:41), would buttress this approach and would help learners and educators alike to manage potentially destructive sex-related and other situations in an intelligent and constructive way.

A new model from Cuba might also help in establishing conditions that would reduce the extent of sexual violence, harassment and abuse to which school pupils are exposed. Cuba is developing lower secondary education provision on the basis of the 'integrated teacher' approach. In this system, one teacher is responsible for teaching all subjects (other than English, computer science and physical education, which have their own specialist teachers) to classes that are deliberately kept small (10 to 15 students). This is similar to the model used in primary schools in the English-speaking Caribbean, but with the added benefit of small class size. The idea is that in this way the teacher will come to know the students intimately and will be able to help and guide them in areas that are wider than what is taught in school. To strengthen the pupil-teacher bonds, the teacher is also required to involve the students' families, through formal weekly meetings and in other ways. In this way it is expected that the teacher will develop a thorough, all-embracing, mentoring relationship with the students, their families and the community. Acts of sexual, physical or verbal violence are probably less likely to occur within a group where this close tripartite relationship involving the teacher, students and parents has been established. The 'integrated teacher' approach cannot, however, be introduced without careful preparation and planning which must include provisions such as Cuba has made for the special training of teachers and the development among them of skills and attitudes that extend beyond mere subject content.

HIV/AIDS brings turmoil into the lives of those whom it affects. The effects impinge very heavily on young people, and even more so when they are socialised in a context where violence is accepted as normal. A major support that schools can provide is to offer them an environment where they will be 'safe from harm, cared for equally and treated with respect' (UNAIDS/UNICEF/WHO, 2002: 35). Education ministries may legislate for this, but in the final analysis it is the schools themselves that must make this safe and supportive environment a reality. The challenge for schools across the Caribbean is to ensure that they do so.

HIV/AIDS education in the workplace

The education sector employs a very large workforce, often the largest in a country. In addition to teachers, there are the numerous officials at central, regional and district levels, their back-up staff, secretaries, general workers, and cleaners. There are also professional, supervisory and support staff, as well as those in examinations councils, curriculum development centres, and other professional units. On the basis of staffing levels elsewhere and pupil-teacher ratios in the Caribbean, a rough estimate of the size of the entire education workforce in the region might be that there is a teacher for every 20 to 30 pupils, a back-up education official or professional for every five teachers, and a general member of staff for every five officials or professionals.

All of these employees are at risk of HIV infection. They all stand in need of ministry guidelines, directives and HIV prevention programmes that will enhance their capacity to avoid infection and enable them to live and function positively, should they be infected or become so. The ministry has a responsibility to itself to provide this support so that it can continue to operate effectively. Equally, it has a responsibility to each of its employees to promote their protection and safety in the face of a life-threatening disease.

Because HIV/AIDS endangers the world of work through its impact on the workforce it is universally recommended that employers establish HIV/AIDS-in-the-workplace training programmes for their staff. 'Employers and their organisations, in consultation with workers and their representatives, should initiate and support programmes at their workplaces to inform, educate and train workers about HIV/ AIDS prevention, care and support and the enterprise's policy on HIV/ AIDS, including measures to reduce discrimination against people infected or affected by HIV/AIDS and specific staff benefits and entitlements' (ILO, 2001: §5.2[c]).

The International Labour Organization (ILO) further recommends that educational programmes take place during paid working hours and course attendance be considered as part of work obligations. The ILO guidelines also pay considerable attention to the programme content, with specific reference to its gender dimension (*Box 12*), and to the training that is needed for peer educators, workers' representatives and others.

It is significant that the ILO also recommends participation by workers, especially those who are HIV positive, in outreach programmes 'within the local community, especially in schools' (ILO, 2001: §6.6). In the spirit of this recommendation, there would be value in education ministries and their sub-units establishing contact with those in industry with a view to promoting the involvement of industrial personnel in activities based in schools and education offices, and the participation of education personnel in activities based in industrial settings. Interactions of this nature would help to break down the barriers of silence and isolation that surround HIV/ AIDS and thereby would make it easier to take the steps needed for HIV prevention, care and support for those infected or affected, and the lessening of negative impacts all round.

Box 12. HIV/AIDS-in-the-workplace: Programmes proposed by the International Labour Organization

Educational programmes

Where practical and appropriate programmes should:

1. Include activities to help individuals assess the risks that face them personally (both as individuals and as members of a group) and reduce these risks through decision-making, negotiation and communication skills, as well as educational, preventative and counselling programmes.

2. Give special emphasis to high-risk behaviour and other risk factors such as occupational mobility that expose certain groups of workers to increased risk of HIV infection.

3. Provide information about transmission of HIV through drug injection and information about how to reduce the risk of such transmission.

4. Enhance dialogue among governments and employers' and workers' organisations from neighbouring countries and at regional level.

5. Promote HIV/AIDS awareness in vocational training programmes carried out by governments and enterprises, in collaboration with workers' organisations.

Box 12 (cont'd).

6. Promote campaigns targeted at young workers and women.

7. Give special emphasis to the vulnerability of women to HIV, and prevention strategies that can lessen this vulnerability (next section).

8. Emphasise that HIV cannot be contracted through casual contact, and that people who are HIV-positive do not need to be avoided or stigmatised, but rather should be supported and accommodated at the workplace.

9. Explain the debilitating effects of the virus and the need for all workers to be empathetic and non-discriminatory towards workers with HIV/AIDS.

10. Give workers the opportunity to express and discuss their reactions and emotions caused by HIV/AIDS.

11. Instruct workers (especially health-care workers) on the use of Universal Precautions (*Box 11*) and inform them of procedures to be followed in case of exposure.

12. Provide education about the prevention and management of STIs and tuberculosis, not only because of the associated risks of HIV infection but also because these conditions are treatable, thus improving workers' general health and immunity.

13. Promote hygiene and proper nutrition.

14. Promote safer sex practices, including instructions on the use of male and female condoms.

15. Encourage peer education and informal education activities.

16. Be regularly monitored, evaluated, reviewed and revised, where necessary.

Gender-specific programmes

1. All programmes should be gender-sensitive, as well as sensitive to race and sexual orientation. This includes targeting women and men, or addressing either women or men in separate programmes, in recognition of the different types and degrees of risk for men and women workers.

Box 12 (cont'd).

2. Information for women needs to alert them to, and explain their higher risk of, infection, in particular the special vulnerability of young women.

3. Education should help both women and men to understand and act upon the unequal power relations between them in employment and personal situations; harassment and violence should be addressed specifically.

4. Programmes should help women to understand their rights, both within the workplace and outside it, and empower them to protect themselves.

5. Education for men should include awareness-raising, risk assessment and strategies to promote men's responsibilities regarding HIV/AIDS prevention.

6. Appropriately targeted prevention programmes should be developed for homosexually active men in consultation with these workers and their representatives.

Source: *An ILO Code of Practice on HIV/AIDS and the World of Work*, International Labour Office, Geneva, 2001, §6.2, 6.3.

Extending and strengthening links between schools and communities

In many societies a large gap exists between the school and community. This is especially so in rural areas. Apart from involvement in the development and maintenance of the school infrastructure, communities often play little part in the life of the school. The role of parents in the actual education of their children may be confined to making the necessary payments, ensuring that the children attend school and do their homework, scrutinising end-of-term reports, and attending relatively infrequent school open days. They are seldom given any more meaningful responsibility. Moreover, in areas where levels of literacy are low, the school may be culturally quite remote from the community, with parents not understanding much that goes on there.

One immediate negative outcome of this is that many students learn at two very distinct levels: the school level, where an analytic, western, urban, individualistic, middle-class approach often prevails; and the community level, where a holistic approach, based on community cohesiveness and rooted in traditional values and beliefs, may predominate. Students straddle two worlds, the proximate and real world of home and community and the more remote and somewhat contrived world of the school. It seems likely that the world of the community will be more influential than the world of the school in shaping values, attitudes, behaviours and practices, including those that protect against the risk of HIV infection. The separation of these two worlds in two fairly water-tight compartments may indeed be part of the reason why school-based HIV/AIDS education does not always lead to responsible, life-protecting sexual behaviour. It is also relevant that, for the greater part, high-risk sexual or drug-injecting behaviours occur mostly in community settings.

These considerations underline the importance of strengthening links between schools and the communities they serve. Both are important in the struggle with HIV/AIDS. The more crucial response must occur at community level. But this needs to be buttressed by the type of institutional support that the school, and only the school, can give.

Education personnel have always been concerned with extending and strengthening the bonds between school and community. HIV/AIDS provides some opportunities for doing this. A general principle is that in the circumstances of the disease, the school should seek to respond to HIV/AIDS needs in the community while the community for its part should seek to respond to HIV/AIDS needs in the school. The triangular model (*Figure 4*) provides a visual representation of the way HIV/AIDS education and concerns can help to promote closer school-community bonds. The majority of the links to be established would be mediated by school learners.

Figure 4. The triangular model for school and community links

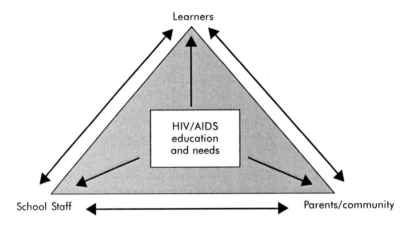

Thus, working closely with communities and parents, the school authorities can:

- arrange for the school community to serve the HIV/AIDS needs of the local community in such areas as participating in home-based care, tending the gardens or animals of those who are sick or caring for the sick, or providing company for the sick or care-givers;

- cooperate with the local community in establishing an environment that is safe – physically, sexually and in drug terms – for school students;

- work with partners in helping communities arrive at a better understanding of HIV/AIDS and how it can be prevented;

- assist communities understand what is meant by life-skills so that they may promote student practice of these skills and thereby contribute to an increase in the levels of harmony and non-violence within a community and a reduction in the levels of high risk behaviours;

- decide jointly with communities on the most appropriate local response to the needs of children infected with HIV, and orphans, and other children made vulnerable by the epidemic.

From the community perspective, parents and members of the local community can:

- agree with the school on the content of the HIV/AIDS messages to be communicated in both school and community settings, so that there is consistency between the messages communicated in the school and those of the home and community;

- participate with the school in the design, and where appropriate in the delivery, of its HIV/AIDS-responsive curriculum;

- assist the school in establishing and running extra-curricular HIV/AIDS-related activities;

- co-operate with the school in providing HIV-infected school members with any special services they need, such as transport to and from school or to medical clinics, or nutritional meals;

- develop with the school the steps both sides need to take to create a school and community environment that is safe, supportive, and non-violent, and that reduces the likelihood of injecting drug use and sexual behaviour which is open to the risk of HIV infection.

HIV/AIDS is everybody's business. Consequently it is important that the entire community be involved on both sides: the whole school community, including student representatives; and the entire local community, including parents and significant local custodians of social values. Because of their role in promoting principles and values, the latter should include religious leaders and those prominent in faith-based organisations. But they should also include others who are important in community and communication circles, such as journalists, musicians, and sports and media personalities.

CHAPTER 6

Preventing HIV/AIDS through Education[1]

Education plays a critical role in the fight against HIV/AIDS. It does so in three complementary ways (*Box 13*). First, it promotes the development of personal value systems and attitudes, backed up by the necessary knowledge and skills, which support individual efforts to remain HIV free. Second, education increases the general capacity of individuals to assimilate information, evaluate situations, and look to future benefits – factors that reduce the likelihood of their engaging in behaviour that carries the risk of HIV infection. Third, it makes a significant contribution to dismantling the ignorance, poverty and disempowerment that singly, and in combination, make men and women more vulnerable to HIV infection.

Box 13. Education's role in preventing HIV infection

In the near term, education provides instruction on HIV prevention and fosters the development of personal knowledge, skills, attitudes and values that support individual efforts to avoid HIV infection and eliminate HIV/AIDS-related stigma.

In the middle term, education promotes general abilities that increase the capacity of the individual to make

---

> ## Box 13 (cont'd).
>
> calculated choices, including the choice to refrain from behaviour that carries the risk of HIV infection.
>
> In the long term, education contributes to society's efforts to eliminate factors that heighten vulnerability to HIV: poverty, ignorance, female disempowerment.

From the near term perspective, education works by providing the learner with understanding of the disease and factors that contribute to risk, laying the foundation for life-skills that can help to keep the individual safe, and demonstrating, in theory and in practice, the case for compassion towards persons infected with or affected by HIV and AIDS. What is important in this immediate sense is what has been learned and how it has been learned. From the middle term perspective, education works by continuing to promote personal efficacy and the sense that one is able to control one's own life. What is important in the middle term is that the individual has been educated to some level. From the long term perspective, education works by transforming society so that conditions favourable to HIV transmission become less dominant. What is important in the long term is the increase in the general level of education in society.

Each of these dimensions is important and education must play its role in all three simultaneously. They do not conflict with one another and are not independent of each other.

Instead, they interpenetrate one another and in general support one another. The long term aspect in improving society and the general effect of education in transforming an individual are crucial components of education's contribution to the struggle against HIV/AIDS. Specific instruction on prevention is of great importance and needs comprehensive attention. But on its own it is not sufficient and almost certainly its beneficial effects are heavily dependent on the success of education in the other two spheres – that of contributing to the transformation of society and that of equipping individuals with a sense of greater efficacy in the control of their lives.

On the other hand, in the circumstances of a world affected by HIV/AIDS, the eradication of poverty; the empowerment of people, especially women and girls; the increase in the levels of tolerance and understanding; and the very characteristic of being in control of one's own life necessitate some understanding of HIV prevention and the steps needed to make it effective. A basic concern in a world with AIDS is that everybody is AIDS-competent – competent enough to prevent personal infection or the transmission of the virus to another person, competent to provide care and support for those infected and affected and to rule out all forms of stigma and discrimination, and competent to mitigate negative impacts within the family and community and across society. This essential AIDS competence is more likely to be achieved if there was more education in general, if each individual was able to access more education, and if more education programmes included specific instruction on HIV/ AIDS and related issues.

Adequate attention to the gender dimension is crucial to all this. In several areas of the world, female disempowerment is a dominant issue. Precisely because they are female, women and girls are treated as if economically and socially subordinate. Failure to educate girls and young women to the same level as boys and young men has accentuated this subordinate status. In its turn, this under-education heightens female vulnerability to sexual exploitation, and hence to exposure to diseases like HIV/AIDS.

In the Caribbean and some developed countries, a different dynamic is at work. Historical and social developments have led to the situation where boys and young men are making less use of educational opportunities than girls and young women. In countries that experience this phenomenon, empowering young males through education is of paramount importance. As noted already in *Chapter 3* above, a major EFA challenge for the Caribbean education sector is to ensure that young males benefit equally with young females from quality education. Likewise, a major HIV/AIDS challenge for the sector is to ensure the active participation of boys and young men in an education-centred response.

These considerations have immediate practical consequences for the greater use of education as a tool for HIV prevention. From the first perspective, efforts should be made to ensure that education programmes incorporate teaching and learning about HIV/AIDS within the context of a healthy lifestyle and on matters that have a bearing on keeping oneself free from HIV infection. From the second perspective, steps should be taken to ensure that every individual has been educated to some basic minimum level. From the third perspective, every effort should be made to raise the general level of education, through the provision of more years of better education.

The World Education Forum (UNESCO, 2000) reaffirmed international commitment to universal primary education as the minimum general level of education for individuals and societies in today's world. While the forum spoke about having access to and completing primary education of good quality, emphasis has shifted to stress the importance of completion, given that those who complete the primary cycle are likely to draw more benefit from their schooling than those who enrol but drop out prematurely. But universal primary education, even with high levels of completion, is only a beginning. Economic prosperity, the reduction of poverty, the realisation in practice of gender equity, and the development of the ability to live together in an atmosphere of tolerance, acceptance and understanding, make it important that increasing proportions of boys and girls enrol in and complete schooling beyond the primary level.

Universal primary completion is already a feature of several Caribbean countries, though not of all. In Haiti, for example, less than half of all children reach the fifth grade (World Bank, 2000: 25). In the English-speaking Caribbean, universal education extends up to age 15 years and in half a dozen countries up to 17 years. In the long term, countries that have extended their systems in this way should find conditions that reduce vulnerability to HIV infection. Hence more vigorous efforts to ensure that all children – especially boys and young men in Caribbean countries – participate in school for several years beyond the primary cycle will, in time, stand to the benefit of these countries in terms of reduced HIV vulnerability.

The evidence is strong that education itself protects against HIV. Young people who are in the process of being educated are less likely to be HIV-infected than their counterparts who are not involved in an education programme. This potential of school education to provide some measure of protection comes out in investigations, conducted in various parts of Africa and in the Caribbean, that show that those who have dropped out of school are more likely to be HIV-infected than those who remain in school. Evidence from Africa shows that girls who had dropped out of school were three times more likely to be HIV-infected than their age-mates who were still attending school. In similar fashion, a case-control study in the Bahamas showed that a significantly higher percentage of women who were HIV-positive were likely to have dropped out of school before age 15 than women in a control group (Stuart and Bain, 1993). A striking feature of these findings is the fact that the education programmes taken by those who were less likely to be HIV-infected included little, if any, formal instruction relating to health skills or HIV/AIDS. What counted for these girls was not so much what they learned but the fact that they were still in an educational programme and had remained in it to a somewhat older age than others.

How participation in an education or training programme works to make a person less likely to become HIV infected is far from being clear. Part of the reason may lie in the way that the better educated person can make more discerning use of information and is better able to evaluate and assimilate information and knowledge (Coombe and Kelly, 2001). In the process of learning, an individual builds up a bank of internal skills for dealing with information sources − analyzing, judging, accepting, rejecting what has been presented. This bank of skills may well be a student's most significant acquisition while in school. Consolidating and extending them is the work of a lifetime. But having acquired them in their most formative years, students retain and subconsciously apply them in all circumstances in life, including those relating to HIV/AIDS and protection-relevant information. In other words, the intellectual skills developed in routine language, social science, mathematics and science programmes stand the learner in good stead subsequently throughout life, enabling the individual to evaluate information and knowledge, in the HIV/AIDS domain as in all others.

It is also the case that the discipline associated with education helps students develop valuable qualities that will influence much of their behaviour in subsequent life. From prolonged experience of the regimented routines and procedures of school, students learn to defer gratification, to apply themselves even when naturally reluctant to do so, to endure constraints and hardships in the expectation of long-term future benefits and to plan for the protection and advancement of their future. In addition, persons with more education tend to have a greater sense of personal efficacy in relation to their own lives, a sense that they are in control and can do something with their lives. They also have a wider range of choices and are better equipped to examine alternatives and make choices that are likely to be to their advantage, including the choice to refrain from behaviour that carries the risk of HIV infection.

It is probably also the case that education as occupation helps keep young people away from situations of risk and from acting out risky behaviour. Opportunities to take major risks do not readily occur when young people have to respond to the educational pressures of class attendance and work on assignments. They do occur in times of relative idleness. The lack of structured occupation, as at weekends and during school holidays, may enable risk-taking on the part of boys and girls, in much the same way as it enables risk-taking on the part of those who do not participate in educational programmes and who are unable to find employment.

These reflections have a clear implication for educational practice. It is that teaching should be of good quality, participative and demanding in its expectations of students. Learners have the potential to develop important affective and intellectual qualities. An education system or programme will promote the development of these qualities if it is well planned, well administered, well taught, and well evaluated.

In other words, the better the quality of education and the more it seeks to promote the total personal development of students, the greater the likelihood that learners will develop attributes that will enhance their personal ability to keep themselves free of HIV infection. Quality education is good in itself. But it is also good at promoting personal attributes that are protective against HIV infection.

The implications of what has been said are that education ministries are already taking action against HIV/AIDS when they:

- promote progress towards universal primary education, in terms of student access, attendance and completion;
- prolong the basic education cycle into an increasing number of years of secondary education;
- ensure excellence in the quality of education programmes, in terms of content, teaching and actual student learning accomplishment;
- ensure that schools have strong administrative leadership that will focus on the quality of instruction, attention to standards of work, and concern for each student.

Most education ministries are likely to agree, however, that they could perform better in what they are already doing. By improving their accomplishments, in terms of access and the quality of learning, they are also improving the potency of their education systems to counter the AIDS epidemic. Attention to expanding access and improving quality is, by the same token, attention to responding positively to HIV/AIDS and preventing infection.

HIV/AIDS in the curriculum

But this is not enough. If it were, no well-educated person would become HIV infected, and this is not the case. There is need also for a purpose-designed educational programme that provides instruction on HIV prevention and fosters the development of personal knowledge, skills, attitudes and values that support individual efforts to avoid HIV infection. The evidence is that this kind of education works in promoting behaviour that reduce the likelihood of HIV infection. 'If preventive education is done right, it is effective. If done immediately, it will have a long-term impact. If done massively, it can turn the tide' (Hernes, 2002: 9).

Caribbean countries, in common with the majority of countries in the world, have sought to integrate sexual and reproductive health (SRH), and life-skills education into the school curriculum. The major benefit reported by countries that have adopted this approach is improved levels of awareness among young people. Better knowledge about AIDS, HIV transmission, prevention and sexuality is clearly a first priority to which education programmes must attend. Information is not sufficient to protect people against HIV infection, but it is a necessary foundation on which prevention efforts must build. It is also fundamental in ensuring respect for the human rights of all who have been affected by the epidemic. Information is of especial importance in settings where sexual activity begins early and measures taken to protect one's sexual health are inadequate. Both of these descriptions apply to many Caribbean countries – see *Box 14* and *Figure 2* on the age of sexual initiation among 10-18 year old school students in nine Caribbean countries. Correct information is of such critical importance that its absence can be lethal, as, for instance, not knowing that HIV can be transmitted through breast milk. Hence there is need to ensure that every young person leaving school, or graduating from an education programme, is well informed on behaviours that carry the risk of HIV infection and those that do not. This information is needed with a view not merely to minimize the risk of HIV transmission, but also to promotehealthy and humane interactions with persons living with HIV/AIDS and countering the stigma and discrimination that so frequently occur.

Box 14. Issues in adolescent sexuality in Jamaica

Trends in sexual activity

- Adolescents engage in early, high-risk activity, with boys starting at an earlier age than girls.

- Most adolescents have sex the first time out of curiosity.

- Boys give physical pleasure and their standing among peers as reasons for having sex.

- Girls are not expected to have premarital pregnancies and feel badly if they do.

- Girls receive mixed messages from family members (especially mothers) about sexual activity and sexuality.

- Men usually offer two main things to get women to have sex with them: money and material things. Sex is expected if a boy spends money on a girl.

- Trading sex for goods and having multiple partners are common among young women.

- For general information about sex, girls under 15 years go to a clinic or friends as their sources. For boys it is peers and relatives.

Sexual health

- Most adolescents feel no risk of contracting HIV/AIDS.

- Older teens, females and inner-city residents are most often affected by sexually transmitted infections.

- Males don't use condoms because they say it spoils their pleasure. Females don't use them if they know their partner well.

- With a non-regular partner, it is the male who decides if a condom is to be used.

- Teachers are the most important source of information on HIV/ AIDS.

Box 14 (cont'd).

- The church is becoming more important as a source of information for boys; schools are more important for girls.

Sexual abuse
- Girls and young women are frequently sexually abused and a first sexual activity often occurs without the girl's consent.
- About 10% of girls and 5% of boys do not feel safe from sexual harassment in the home.

Source: Meeting Adolescent Development and Participation Rights, UNICEF/UNFPA, Kingston, 2002: 3.

In Caribbean countries, the HIV prevalence rates among young people aged 15-24 are high and in some instances may be considerably higher than the rates among the wider population aged 15-49 (*Table 4*). This situation holds great significance for the future of the region. It also suggests that school based initiatives may not yet have had any significant influence on the behaviour patterns of students. It seems likely that this may be because the Health and Family Life Education (HFLE) initiative, the flagship health education programme of the Caribbean Community (CARICOM), which is described below, is still getting under way.

Table 4. HIV prevalence rates among young people (15-24) in selected Caribbean countries, 2001

	Adult prevalence rate (15-49)	Estimated range of prevalence rates among young people (15-24)	
	All (%)	Female (%)	Male (%)
Bahamas	3.5	2.0-4.1	1.7-36
Barbados*	1.2	0.8-0.9	1.0-1.4
Belize	2.0	1.6-2.4	0.9-1.3
Cuba	<0.1	0.0-0.1	0.1-0.1
Dominican Republic	2.5	2.2-3.3	1.7-2.5
Guyana	2.7	2.6-5.4	2.1-4.4
Haiti	6.1	3.2-6.7	2.6-5.5
Jamaica	1.2	0.7-1.0	0.7-1.0
Trinidad & Tobago	2.5	2.1-4.4	1.6-3.3

Source: *Report on the Global HIV/AIDS Epidemic*, UNAIDS. 2002*a*. Data for Barbados from the June 2000 edition of the Report.

The health and family life education programme

The HFLE initiative is a life-skills based programme that fosters the development of the knowledge, skills and attitudes that make for healthy personal, family and social life. The aim of the programme is to help children and young people understand that the choices they make in everyday life profoundly influence their health and personal development into adulthood and to persuade them to practice healthy choices. Areas covered include health and well-being, nutrition, eating and fitness, human sexuality and sexual health (including HIV infection and AIDS), self development and interpersonal relationships, substance abuse, and managing the environment.

In 1996, the document *Strategy for Strengthening Health and Family Life Education in CARICOM States* received the approval in principle of policy-makers as well as HFLE specialists in CARICOM countries. This plan of action focuses on four major areas:

- Policy measures to raise the status of HFLE at all levels of the educational system.
- Improvement of HFLE facilitator and teacher training.
- Development of comprehensive life-skills based materials for HFLE.
- Strengthening coordination among institutions engaged in HFLE at national ands regional levels.

At the time of writing, approved or draft policies have been developed in ten countries. Regional training programmes have been provided for cross-sectoral country teams (representing education, health, and community development) and these in turn are responsible for the conduct of in-country training activities. In some countries, teachers in primary and secondary schools have been oriented to HFLE, some of them to specialist level. Increasing emphasis has been placed on ensuring the inclusion of HFLE in the curriculum of teacher training institutions, while discussions are on-going about including HFLE as a core subject for initial teacher certification. A needs assessment study has been carried out in nine countries to determine the current implementation of HFLE in schools and to obtain a better understanding of needs and expectations of the main target groups. The process has been initiated of developing HFLE curriculum outlines for pre-primary, primary and secondary schools, as well as classroom materials to support the teaching of HFLE in schools. In terms of co-ordination, national HFLE committees that seek to co-ordinate national HFLE activities operate in several countries, while a regional HFLE working group (with representatives from the UN agencies, UWI School of Education, and CARICOM) meets at least once a year to review and plan for regional HFLE activities.

The FRESH initiative

It is clear that much has been done to lay the groundwork for the successful implementation of the HFLE concept. Since the HFLE idea was first mooted in the early 1990s, the global community has committed itself to creating safe, healthy, inclusive and equitably resourced educational environments conducive to excellence in learning and clearly defined levels of achievement for all. To this end a new global initiative, Focusing Resources on Effective School Health (FRESH), was launched at the World Education Forum held in Dakar in April 2000. The FRESH approach is based on two understandings: first, that the goal of universal education cannot be achieved while the health needs of children and adolescents go unmet; and second, that a core group of cost effective activities can be implemented, together and in all schools, in order to meet these needs.

The core framework of action for the FRESH initiative consists of four components that should be made available together in all schools:

- *Health-related school policies* that would look to ensuring a safe and secure physical environment and a positive psycho-social school culture and would address issues such as the abuse of students, sexual harassment, substance abuse, family life education, the further education of girls who become pregnant, and attitudes towards people with HIV/AIDS and their families.

- *Provision of safe water and adequate sanitation in schools*, as an essential first step towards a healthy learning environment.

- *Skills-based health education* that would seek to develop the knowledge, attitudes, values, and life-skills needed to make, and act on, the most appropriate and positive health-related decisions, so as to reduce the number of unwanted pregnancies and dropouts from school, address lack of knowledge about HIV/AIDS and reduce risk behaviour, reduce short-term hunger and improve nutrition, and reduce substance abuse.

- *School-based health and nutrition services*, such as responding to micronutrient deficiencies and worm infections, providing school snacks, or changing the time of meals.

Clearly, there are many areas of potential overlap between the FRESH and HFLE initiatives. If the HFLE programme were implemented in all schools of the region, with adequate attention to the kind of skills-based health education proposed in the previous paragraph, facilitator and teacher training in these areas, and the development of classroom materials, it might be regarded as the Caribbean's unique contribution to the debate. The Regional Strategic Plan of Action for HIV/AIDS includes support for the implementation of the programme among its strategic objectives and identifies the activities needed to achieve this objective (*Box 15*).

Box 15. Key activities for the implementation of the HFLE programme

1. Identify and address main obstacles to the effective implementation of the HFLE programme.

2. Review existing curricula and promote inclusion of improved materials on HIV and STIs.

3. Develop and implement the necessary policy directives that will ensure the implementation of HFLE programmes and other adolescent friendly activities at national level.

4. Include National AIDS Programmes in multisectoral HFLE committees.

5. Assess needs for and availability of adolescent friendly health services in the region

Source: The Caribbean Regional Strategic Plan of Action for HIV/AIDS.

There would be reason, therefore, to seek to draw into the HFLE initiative international resources that might be available for the implementation of the FRESH programme and to use these resources to revitalize HFLE from a FRESH perspective, with universalization of its coverage and its firm insertion into teacher education programmes. A revitalized FRESH-inspired HFLE programme should be able to build on the political support that HFLE has already attracted. The next step would be for FRESH and HFLE specialists in the region to work together for the comprehensive and effective implementation of a unified programme. In the context of HIV/AIDS, such a unified programme would have great potential to address the need for basic information, clear understanding, essential skills, and a rights-based approach.

Learning from elsewhere

Experience with school-based HIV/AIDS and reproductive health programmes in other parts of the world suggests the importance of the following dimensions:

- *The curriculum approach* needs to identify HIV/AIDS, sexual and reproductive health (SRH) and life-skills education as a sphere of knowledge and understanding that constitutes a professional subject area in its own right, with a dedicated corps of educators and teacher educators – from university down to school level – who are the specialized professionals in this field.

- *The curriculum design* should ensure that HIV/AIDS, SRH and life-skills education is not spread thinly across a number of carrier subjects, but is coherently embedded as a stand-alone area within the curriculum. This subject area enhances the likelihood that children and young people will live. Hence it deserves as much prominence as subjects such as mathematics and English that prepare children and young people for life. Moreover, the all-important links with broader health education programmes and readily available, youth-friendly and adequately resourced health services should be stressed (IATT, 2002: 22-26).

- *The teaching methodology* should make provision for peer teaching, approaches such as Process Drama that give scope to emotional and affective expression, the participation of parents and communities, the involvement of persons living with HIV/AIDS, and participation by religious and other community leaders. There should be less reliance on whole-class teaching in formal settings. In addition, the weight of the evidence suggests the inadvisability of HIV/AIDS, SRH and life-skills becoming a formal examination subject. In-class programmes should be supported by required extra-curricular activities. Ideally, these would include the provision of services to families affected by HIV/AIDS.

- *Teachers should be given the help they need* so that they feel adequately prepared to teach this area. This necessitates attention to boosting their knowledge and understanding, helping them to deal with sensitive, and in some cases taboo topics, and making them able to deal comfortably with a life and death issue which may be very close to home for some of them. Initial professional training to work as teachers of HIV/ AIDS, SRH and life-skills needs to be supported by ongoing training that will respond to the intellectual and the special emotional or affective needs that teachers in this area may experience.

- *The work in schools should be supported by adequate, scientifically accurate, good quality teaching and learning materials.* There should also be provision for the backup, guidance, teacher support structures, monitoring and evaluation that other subjects receive. *The Strategic Framework on HIV/AIDS and Education*, produced by the Inter-Agency Task Team (IATT), highlights various areas where teachers may need special support and preparation – 'for issues of confidentiality; identifying and making better use of resources outside educational institutions, including medical, psychological, social and other services; in helping access counselling, care and prevention; in supporting colleagues and students; and in coping with their own emotional and physical needs' (IATT, 2002: 33).

The objective of preventive education programmes

The ultimate objective of education's concern in the area of HIV prevention should be to promote behaviour that will not put an individual or any partner at risk of infection. For many young people, this will involve helping them to maintain safe, existing behavioural patterns. For others it will involve helping them to replace behavioural patterns and activities that put them at risk of HIV infection with those that are safe. Placing the emphasis on maintaining existing, risk-free behaviour patterns accords well with the fact that the majority of adults and young people do not become HIV infected and hence may not need to change their behaviour. It also expresses more confidence in the ability and commitment of the majority of adults and young people to behave in a sexually responsible way.

Hence the thrust of educational efforts to stem HIV transmission should be to empower those who participate in programmes to live sexually responsible, healthy lives. This implies understanding, leading to practice, in two areas, healthy sexuality and healthy living. These are the two principal areas around which programmes should be developed. They are central to everything else, and from them must flow the values and attitudes that will manifest themselves in information, practices, skills, and techniques.

This means that in the context of the sexual transmission of HIV, a good preventive programme will begin at the proper beginning, that is, in promoting a balanced understanding of sexuality and relationships. Educators should not hesitate to affirm that both of these are very good and beautiful. They should help learners to appreciate the wonderful, extremely powerful energy of sexuality, experienced in every cell of one's being, as a mighty urge to overcome incompleteness and to find fulfilment in a strong and abiding relationship with another person, of the same or opposite sex. Recognising the special importance of relationships for adolescents and young adults, educators should be equally forceful in affirming the value of a relationship that needs safeguards, whether these consist of no sex, deferred sex, or protected sex.

Having sex – or genitality, the physical, genital dimension of sexuality – is a very important aspect of these larger realities of sexuality and relationships. But it is no more than an aspect. It does not exhaust the full notion of sexuality which can work powerfully and constructively even in the absence of the particularised, physical, often short-lived bodily encounter with another that constitutes 'having sex'. In practical terms this means that it would be a mistake for an educator to focus on protection messages, whether these relate to abstinence, condom use or delaying sexual debut, prior to establishing a good understanding of the meaning of sexuality and relationships. Too often, preventive education programmes focus too early on the knowledge, attitudes and skills involved in immediate, physical sexual practice, without striving to embed these in a more holistic approach that takes account of the roots of human behaviour. It is not surprising, then, to find that the desired practices may be maintained as long as the programmes last, but do not persist when the programmes end.

The second basic area for consideration is healthy living. Conditions of poverty facilitate HIV transmission partly because the body's defence mechanisms are already run down through malnutrition, the legacy of other illnesses, a heavy burden of parasites (especially from malaria), and vitamin and trace element deficiency. When HIV succeeds in gaining admission to such an impoverished body its task is greatly facilitated. The individual can become infected in circumstances where a better nourished and healthier individual would be able to ward off the infection. Increasing attention to host susceptibility to HIV infection is opening new avenues for understanding the spread of the virus and for the design of effective prevention strategies (Stillwaggon, 2000). What is emerging clearly is that maintaining a healthy way of living, including paying attention to basic personal hygiene and adhering to a balanced diet using available foods, is in itself a substantial step in the direction of preventing HIV infection.

It is also worth noting that school curricula, which used to include teaching children the principles and practice of personal and environmental hygiene, appear to have gone out of use. There is a case for restoring these topics, so that children can be taught systematically how to care for their bodies and for the environment around them. The FRESH initiative could accommodate this area without adding to curriculum overload.

Healthy living is also a significant step in the direction of slowing down the progression from HIV to clinical AIDS. All other things being equal, infected persons who maintain a healthy life style are likely to enjoy more years of life than infected persons who do not take balanced nourishing meals, who smoke, take alcohol or use drugs, and who do not take adequate exercise and rest.

The content of a comprehensive preventive education programme

Ideally, the content of a comprehensive HIV prevention programme, whether delivered through schools or otherwise, should extend to the following areas:

- Sexuality and relationships, leading to a good understanding of what sexuality means, its role in relationships, and the norms for a healthy sexuality.

- Manifesting respect and regard for others in a spirit of equality and power-sharing between males and females that extends to all areas of life.

- Knowledge and understanding of HIV/AIDS, the modes of transmission, what infection does within the human body, how it progresses, and how it can be treated.

- Popular misconceptions, errors and myths relating to HIV/ AIDS.

- A core set of psycho-social life-skills for the promotion of the health and well-being of learners. These should include self-respect and self-care, decision-making, interpersonal relationships, self-awareness, stress and anxiety management, coping with pressures, conflict negotiation, assertiveness, and the development of self-esteem and self-confidence.

- Knowledge and understanding of how to manage and protect one's reproductive health.

- The role and value of abstinence, the development of positive attitudes towards this, and the skills that enable one to abstain from sexual activity.
- HIV risk-reducing factors, such as delayed sexual debut, reducing the frequency of partner exchange, avoidance of casual sex or the management of such encounters to protect against HIV transmission.
- Fidelity in marriage and the management of marriage relationships where HIV is present.
- The meaning of protected sex, the role it plays in preventing HIV infection, the skills that are implied, and how to access and use condoms and other supplies.
- The desirability of voluntary counselling and testing, and the importance of early presentation of sexually transmitted infections (STIs) to the appropriate health services.
- The risk of HIV infection associated with alcohol or drug consumption and injecting drug use.
- The meaning of a healthy lifestyle, its role in making an individual less susceptible to HIV infection, and its role in promoting the quality of life and extending the survival years of an individual who is HIV infected.

Some observations need to be addressed about this comprehensive programme. First, learners should be introduced to it while they are still very young – some would say from the day they commence school. While it may be necessary to begin at a later age for those who are already in the school system, HIV/AIDS-related forms of education should start as early as possible with younger children, and certainly well before they enter the period of puberty. This means that pupils should be introduced to HIV preventive education no later than middle primary school. Even earlier would be better. Later would be too late. But whatever is presented to children must be appropriate to their age and grade. It would be foolhardy and counterproductive to expose young children to matters that were beyond their comprehension and experience.

Second, there is a need to remain sensitive to the concerns of parents and community leaders. These may express the fear that some elements in the programme that has been outlined might lead learners to increased sexual behaviour and experimentation. They need to be reassured that the overwhelming weight of evidence is that this form of education does not lead to an explosion in sexual activity. On the contrary, careful investigations, in developing and developed countries alike, have found that it contributes to delay in the onset of sexual activity, increased recourse to abstinence, reduction in the number of sexual partners, and a lessening of the incidence of STIs and unwanted pregnancies (Gachuhi, 1999; UNAIDS, 1997). Open discussion with the representatives of parents, and with cultural, traditional and religious leaders, can help to ensure that the messages are communicated within a framework that accords with the best values from these traditions. The participation of these groups in the actual communication process may well be one of the best ways of ensuring that significant parties are all speaking with one voice, a factor that is crucial to the translation of programme messages into practice.

The importance of both these aspects was underlined by UNAIDS in its 1999 World AIDS Campaign with Children and Young People:

> Policies on integrating quality life-skills, sexual health, and HIV/AIDS education into school curricula, **starting at primary school** and continuing throughout a student's education, must be developed by Ministries of Education, **in collaboration with parent-teacher associations and with the participation of** student representatives. ... In addition it is critical that children and young people who do not attend school are also given access to life-skills, sexual health and HIV/AIDS training (UNAIDS, 1999a: 17).

Third, the approach, the materials and the presentations should strive to be positive and confident. In the early days of the HIV/AIDS epidemic, many communication programmes sought to induce fear, believing that this would lead to the maintenance or adoption of risk-free sexual behaviour. But experience has shown that scare tactics do not work. Neither do lists of prohibitions that are not rooted in understanding of the issues. These may be easy to formulate, but they do not adequately provide young people with guidance on how to act or behave. The avoidance of defeatism is also important. People are already sufficiently weighed down by the magnitude of HIV/AIDS. Young people sense this. They do not need to have the burden increased. Instead they need to be enthused with a vision of the world in which the epidemic will be overcome. They need to be encouraged to develop a strong conviction that it is they who will secure this victory through their own life-styles, as they take ownership of the issues and drive a youth-centred response.

Speaking with one voice

In conclusion, it cannot be stressed too strongly that, if HIV preventive education programmes are to be effective, there should be no conflicting messages. Conflict and lack of unanimity lead to confusion and lack of action.

The sexual transmission of HIV occurs through behaviour that takes place in very private circumstances. It is also behaviour that is deeply instinctual, giving physical expression to what is probably the most basic and powerful of human energies. Advocacy to modify, shape or change that behaviour is not always welcome. However, it may be effective if the content of the messages is consistently the same. It stands a considerable chance of being ignored if conflicting messages are received. Thus, if one group advocates condom use while another group decries this as immoral, or if one group advocates abstinence while another group disparages this as impossible, the effect will be to leave individuals not knowing what they should do. And in such circumstances the majority will continue to behave in the way they always did.

Senegal and Uganda have shown a better way forward. They agreed to sink differences by approving a common menu of approaches from which every group could choose whatever best fitted in with its philosophy and ideology, and agreeing to stay silent about approaches that caused misgiving or offence. In no case did any group belittle or condemn the approach adopted by others. This allowed government, civil society, traditional leaders, and faith organisations to convey non-conflicting messages, a fact that is believed to have made a very positive contribution to the success of these countries. In fact Senegal in containing the spread of HIV while Uganda is rolling back prevalence rates.

In several countries people have become so confused about AIDS – where it originated, what causes it, how it can be prevented – that they have ceased to hear the messages that are being conveyed. In their suffering they are crying out for clarity and unanimity from their teachers and leaders. Every educator is duty bound to ensure that they are answered appropriately and that the answers are not in conflict with one another. The sufferings of people, the cry of the poor, and the future of much of the human race demand no less.

Notes

1.   In addition to the material contained in this and subsequent chapters, useful guidelines are provided in the booklet Preventing HIV/AIDS in Schools (Schenker and Nyirenda, 2002) which can be freely downloaded from www.ibe.unesco.org/publications, or can be obtained free on request from the International Bureau of Education (IBE), Geneva.

CHAPTER 7

Managing the Education Sector Response to HIV/AIDS

The challenge to provide leadership

The HIV/AIDS epidemic constitutes a major threat to the education agenda at global, regional and national levels. It makes it more difficult to attain desirable educational goals. It confronts the sector with complex and demanding situations that challenge its ability to provide meaningful, relevant educational services of acceptable quality. It produces new challenges that require bold and creative responses. Issues and problems are recognised more readily in countries that are experiencing high HIV prevalence levels. But they are not confined to these. They can also be experienced in countries where the overall prevalence rates are relatively low but where high prevalence occurs in concentrated pockets, among certain severely infected sectors of the population.

The implications for education management are simple but profound:

1. In its efforts to provide and, where necessary, expand quality education and training, the education system must be managed so that it takes account of HIV/AIDS.

2. Notwithstanding the actual or potential adverse impacts of HIV/ AIDS, the system must be managed in such a way that it continues to function satisfactorily at central, local and institutional levels.

Universal experience with the epidemic during its first two decades has been that such HIV/AIDS-oriented management will be provided only if there is a climate of committed and informed leadership. Strong leadership in every sector is essential for an effective response to the epidemic. Within the education sector it is the essential foundation on which the sector's response must be built. In the circumstances of HIV/AIDS, it is not sufficient that education leaders be adequate or even good (*Box 16*). It is necessary that they be great!

Leadership is the capacity to effect change by inspiring other people to become involved, effective, and, often, enthusiastic in doing what needs to be done. It is based on knowledge of a situation, commitment to act in relation to that situation, willingness to manifest that commitment publicly, willingness to commit personal resources (including time and energy) to the situation, ability to provide personal example and encouragement, and preparedness to work with and through others, showing confidence in their contribution and making allowances for their different perspectives.

To be really effective, leadership must be well informed. There is need for recognition that the situation is grave and structures are under threat. Hence, in the education sector, the first requirement is that the minister, other political leaders, and senior education staff know about HIV/AIDS and its actual or potential impacts. For many, this will necessitate learning more about the interaction between HIV/AIDS and education.[1] For all, it will involve keeping up-to-date on the progress of the epidemic, its impacts on education and the responses coming from the education sector in their own country and elsewhere. There can be no substitute for good information. Resources dedicated to ensuring deep understanding of the epidemic on the part of the political, administrative and professional leaders are resources well spent.

Box 16. Leaders – adequate, good and great

Leadership of a special kind is being tested today. There are those who honestly manage the day-to-day tasks of their institutions and governments. These are adequate leaders.

Other leaders do more. They spend time inspiring people to be better than they otherwise would be, and to act not only for their own selfish ends but for the benefit of all. These are good leaders.

Then there are leaders who rise to face unusual threats to their people. They search for answers and successes, and when they find them, they scale up the response to the maximum. They surpass even themselves, mustering the energies of the whole people. They crusade for change and reform. And they lead by personal example as well as by exhortation. They are selfless. They are dedicated. And they do everything they can to bring success to their people. They are the great leaders. They are the leaders who will be remembered.

Source: K. Y. Amoako, Executive Secretary, Economic Commission for Africa, in Address to African Development Forum 2000, AIDS: The Great Leadership Challenge, Addis Ababa, December 2000.

The second requirement for effective leadership is personal commitment, arising in the case of education from a better understanding of what HIV/AIDS can do to education and what education, for its part, can do to HIV/AIDS. In practical terms this requires that the minister and all senior ministry personnel put their full weight behind the sector's struggle with HIV/AIDS, use the best available human resources in the strategic areas of prevention, care and impact mitigation, and demonstrate through sustained and public communications that, until it has been overcome, HIV/AIDS remains at the core of the education agenda. This commitment will manifest itself by:

- developing policies and strategies that respond to the impact of the epidemic on the sector and to the evolving HIV/AIDS situation;
- ensuring extensive and recurring advocacy, sensitisation and publicity campaigns;
- making the decisions and ensuring the resources that are needed for the implementation of HIV/AIDS pledges and undertakings;
- establishing and staffing any HIV/AIDS-related structures that may be needed, even at the expense of other operations; and
- monitoring the HIV-related activities of those responsible for coordination, curriculum and materials, information gathering and dissemination, planning, and training.

Acting out this commitment may require courageous decisions, such as:

- revisiting education policies and plans, even in their global conception, to ensure that they are fully HIV/AIDS compliant;
- re-examining the very structures of educational provision to ensure that they extend in practice and principle to those infected or affected by the disease (and hence ensuring, for example, that no HIV/AIDS-related circumstance will obstruct the full educational participation of orphans or other children whom the disease has made vulnerable);
- insisting that schools and teachers provide age-appropriate HIV/ AIDS education, as well as sexual and reproductive health education, for all learners;
- ensuring that initial and ongoing teacher preparation programmes incorporate HIV/AIDS, sexual and reproductive health education, and training in life-skills as basic components;

- making absolutely sure that every level of the sector shows zero tolerance for HIV/AIDS-related stigma or discrimination;

- ensuring that those living with HIV/AIDS – be they learners, teachers or other education personnel – can continue to learn or work within the sector, with as much support as can be provided, for as long as they are able.

Extending knowledge on the interaction between HIV/AIDS and education in Caribbean countries

There is an urgent need for more and better information on the interaction between HIV/AIDS and education. Not enough is known as yet about the ways in which the epidemic affects systems and how systems are responding to its impacts. The secrecy, silence and denial so frequently associated with the disease play a significant role in making it difficult to get a clear picture. But in addition it must be recognised that this is a comparatively new area of investigation. It was only in the latter years of the twentieth century that education ministries and international bodies began to address themselves to the potency of the epidemic to undermine education and other systems. Significant advances were made in a short space of time. Nevertheless there are still many information and knowledge gaps. There is much anecdotal information but only a very limited amount of well-conceived and diligently executed empirical research.

Of particular concern to Caribbean countries is the fact that very little is known about the interaction between HIV/AIDS and education in countries where HIV prevalence levels are comparatively low. In severely affected countries, such as Haiti or many of the countries of Africa, it is possible to infer that there will be certain impacts. But even in some of these cases, decisions are being made on the basis of inferences and surmises and not necessarily on the basis of hard, empirical evidence. In low prevalence countries, the foundation hardly exists for such surmises. It is probably fair to say that if the prevalence levels in these countries increases to what it is in Haiti or the African countries, then the adverse impacts on educational provision and quality will very likely be similar. To avoid this, as well as the other disastrous impacts of the epidemic on human beings and systems, low prevalence countries should orient their education systems as strongly as possible to prevention education. In their circumstances this would seem to be the highest priority.

But even low prevalence countries need better information on such matters as:

- the extent of the epidemic within the sector and its institutions;
- its extent within communities served by the sector;
- the impacts the epidemic may already be having on individuals, communities and the system;
- how these impacts affect the core functions of education;
- whether the epidemic is becoming greater or less within the sector;
- how affected educators, learners and communities are coping;
- the responses that are being made by institutions and their leaders;
- the extent to which human resources within the sector have been affected;
- the impacts, if any, on the financial resources for the sector; and
- the nature, extent and source of the support given to learners or educators affected by the epidemic.

It is acknowledged that some important factors may make it difficult for low prevalence countries in the Caribbean to document all of these issues. Assembling good information can be impeded by practices of confidentiality, low levels of HIV testing, and inadequate legal frameworks (for instance, in some Caribbean countries, HIV is not a notifiable disease). Nevertheless, it is only on the basis of this and similar information that education ministries can come to a good understanding of the problem, precisely as it affects them. Likewise, it is only on the basis of this understanding that they can plan for dealing with the problem. Hence there is need to try to overcome the obstacles so as to extend the information base needed for adequate management and planning responses to the epidemic.

This points to the need for systematic investigations that specifically address the actual and likely impacts of HIV/AIDS on educational provision in each country. Although there is a rich body of research in Caribbean countries on issues such as gender and sexual development, information and understanding in the area of HIV/AIDS and education is much more limited. A critical need, therefore, is for education ministries to conduct or commission impact studies that will analyse the situation, analyse the responses that are already under way, and advise on strategies and implementation plans that would strengthen education's response. The example of Haiti, which has led the way in conducting such a study (Haiti, 2002), is worthy of emulation. Although the scale of the epidemic is many times greater in African countries, and the socio-economic environment is very different, impact assessments that are being designed for Caribbean countries could learn from those conducted in some African countries, notably those from Swaziland (Swaziland Ministry of Education, 1999), South Africa (Abt Associates, 2001), and Botswana, Malawi and Uganda (Bennell et al., 2002).

SWOT analysis and rapid appraisal

An impact assessment should help an education ministry identify the key issues that it really needs to address if it is to be successful in minimising the impact of HIV on the sector and maximising the impact of education on the epidemic. But even in the absence of such an assessment, while waiting for its results, or as an integral component of its strategic planning process (*Figure 4*), the ministry can make use of other techniques to expand its understanding of how HIV/AIDS is affecting the sector and what it should do in response. A familiar and easily applied technique, a SWOT analysis. Less well known is the Rapid Appraisal Framework. This is significant for its power in enabling an education ministry to assess the progress it is making in responding to the impact of HIV/AIDS on the sector.

A SWOT analysis examines the strengths, weaknesses, opportunities and threats that arise because of HIV/AIDS in the education sector. The strengths and weaknesses look internally at the ministry and where, in relation to the presence of the epidemic in the sector and community, the ministry is taking action or has the capacity to do so, and likewise where it is inactive, ineffective or lacks capacity. The opportunities and threats look externally at the epidemic as it manifests in society. The threats it poses for an education ministry in an individual country can usually be identified without much difficulty. Identifying opportunities can be a greater problem and some might ask how a development disaster such as HIV/AIDS could present promising opportunities. But the conviction is growing throughout the world that precisely because of its scale and crisis dimensions AIDS demands that many things previously taken for granted be re-visited and re-thought. In particular, it presents a unique opportunity to reconsider many areas in the educational sphere that stand in need of reform (Afterword).

A well-conducted SWOT analysis is likely to identify key issues that the ministry should address in relation to the epidemic. It may also point in the direction of key strategic interventions. It works best if inputs come not just from the ministry's management team, but also from sub-groups within the ministry, on the basis of their specific professional expertise or common interest, and also from groups representing teachers, parents, and civic or community organizations that are linked to the education sector.

The Rapid Appraisal Framework (*Appendix 2*) presents a set of questions that probe whether the education sector, faced with HIV/AIDS, has equipped itself to maintain an adequate and acceptable quality of educational provision. It asks about the extent to which a foundation for action has been laid in terms of policy, leadership, commitment, planning and resource mobilization; whether suitable management structures exist to guide a response; how well prepared educators are to respond to the epidemic; the extent of awareness and advocacy activities; and the research agenda and information needs in relation to HIV/AIDS and education.

This simple tool can be used in a variety of ways, for instance, to:

- help education sector personnel appreciate the range of HIV/AIDS impact issues;
- guide and support the work of HIV/AIDS facilitators;
- guide strategic planning;
- help evaluate action plans; and
- provide guidelines for monitoring and evaluation.

Zero budget planning

The misconception exists that AIDS-related interventions are necessarily costly in terms of the time that must be spent in their preparation, the skills needed for strategic planning, and the resources needed for their implementation. This is not always the case. There are several valuable interventions that can be made without recourse to strategic plans, a ministry's budget, or external funding. There are activities that can be undertaken on a zero budget basis. They may cost something in terms of time for actual implementation, but they have virtually no financial implications. Zero budget planning consists essentially of a brainstorming session, within a ministry, one of its sections, or one of its institutions, to determine worthwhile actions that can be taken on a professional or personal basis. *Box 17* shows some zero budget interventions proposed by education officials in other parts of the world, but it would be up to Caribbean educators to determine for themselves which interventions, costing virtually nothing in financial terms, could be of importance.

Box 17. Zero budgeting

HIV/AIDS-related education interventions that can be implemented immediately and at minimal financial cost:

- Include something about HIV/AIDS in school assemblies, at staff meeting, meetings with parents, meetings of school governors, etc.
- Have HIV/AIDS messages printed on education stationery (exercise books, folders, etc.).
- Hold debates, essay and other competitions on HIV/AIDS topics, with red ribbon awards.
- Invite entertainers, sports personalities and individuals respected by students to talk about HIV/AIDS.
- Invite persons living with HIV/AIDS (PLAs) to address school gatherings.
- Provide for inclusion of HIV/AIDS issues in co-curricular activities.
- Use school drama, school magazines, and school open days to communicate HIV/AIDS messages.
- Establish HIV/AIDS committees at both school and ministry levels.
- Organise individual or class project work with an HIV/AIDS focus.

Prioritising objectives and activities

It is almost always necessary for education officials to prioritize objectives and actions. There may be many directions that promise good progress, but it is not always possible to embark on all of them simultaneously. Moreover, changing external circumstances may mean either the impossibility of doing all that was planned or the possibility of doing more than was expected. A clear sense of priorities will enable managers to respond to such circumstances and make the necessary choices.

General criteria for priorities are that an objective or work activity should be chosen in areas with the greater need, where the impact is likely to be greater, or where there is likely to be a multiplier effect. More specifically, the following criteria can be used to guide prioritization:

- the activity reaches the biggest number;
- the activity promises to make the maximum impact on a specific aspect of the epidemic;
- the activity addresses the most urgent challenge (for instance, by targeting the most vulnerable children);
- the activity promises the maximum leverage, making the biggest impact for the smallest effort, and promising quick and visible positive results;
- the activity is in an area that nobody else is addressing;
- implementation is straightforward because the activity will use existing processes and infrastructure;
- the activity is independent and can be executed without conditionalities or other prerequisite activities;
- the activity is prerequisite to other important interventions;
- the activity being considered is not controversial, but will easily get the necessary political, professional and administrative commitment;
- the activity uses locally available resources that facilitate immediate implementation.

A framework for action

In order to manage its response to HIV/AIDS in the sector, an education ministry needs a framework for action. A comprehensive framework embraces structures, activities and partnerships, all of which help the ministry to think, plan and act more systematically on HIV/AIDS issues.

Structures

In accordance with perceived need, certain structures need to be established at the top political level, at the central ministry level, and at lower levels. The purpose of such structures would be to ensure that HIV/AIDS remains high on the agenda and that there are designated officers – full-time appointees, if the needs are sufficiently great – who would be responsible for the development of proposals and the implementation of decisions.

This could entail one or more of the following:

1. Appointing a special HIV/AIDS advisor to the minister.

2. Creating a focal point within the central ministry, with responsibility for coordinating and maintaining the momentum of ministry programmes and activities; gathering, maintaining and disseminating information on the programmes and activities of every player in the field (the ministry, NGOs, faith-based organizations, international partner agencies, etc.); monitoring and evaluating programmes and activities; ensuring the development, production and dissemination of materials; and ensuring the sensitisation of all ministry staff on HIV/AIDS (through AIDS-in-the-workplace or similar programmes).

3. Establishing a National Task Force for HIV/AIDS-in-Education, with representation from the education and health ministries, other relevant government bodies, NGOs, faith-based organisations, teacher unions, parents, the media, civic leaders, persons living with HIV/ AIDS, the National AIDS Council or Programme, and international partner agencies.

4. Establishing HIV/AIDS-in-Education Committees at national and all sub-national administrative levels (province, district, etc.) and in every institution.

5. Establishing contact points in ministry headquarters, and in all lower level offices, where employees can make confidential contact with management on their HIV status.

Activities

Working at the sectoral level with and through other branches of the ministry, and at the multisectoral level with other government ministries, the international community, NGOs and other organs of civil society, the focal point in the education ministry should ensure that activities are undertaken in the areas of advocacy and sensitisation; coordination; curriculum and materials; information and networking; monitoring, evaluation and research; orphans and vulnerable children; planning; policies and procedures; publicity; school activities; training for capacity building; and youth friendly health services. In these areas (presented alphabetically), plans should be drawn up for specific activities, along the lines suggested below.

Advocacy and sensitisation

- Hold national and lower-level/parish HIV/AIDS-in-Education Conferences:
  - for the public,
  - for teachers/educators.
- Hold information, advocacy, planning workshops for parents, teachers, educators, students in all educational sub-districts, in every teacher education institution, and for every school and college governing body.
- Promote action-based research in colleges and schools to identify households in distress, and provide these with support (as part of co-curricular activities) through home-based care, assistance with income-generating activities, education provided by college and school students to out-of-school children in their homes, etc.
- Make extensive use of the resources inherent in persons living with HIV/AIDS for various advocacy and sensitisation activities.
- Promote the participation of entertainment and media personalities in advocacy and sensitisation activities.

Coordination

- Develop and maintain a living matrix of partners, programmes, interventions, and studies being undertaken by the ministry, NGOs, FBOs, international agencies, etc.
- Promote interaction and the sharing of information and experiences by everyone active in the field of HIV/AIDS and education.
- Gather and disseminate information on interventions that work and those that do not.

Curriculum and materials

- Facilitate discussion by educators, communities (including religious and civic leaders) and young people, on HIV/AIDS, sexual and reproductive health (SRH) and HFLE programmes (and materials) for every school grade (from the first grade onwards) and for every level of teacher education.
- Facilitate curriculum specialists in the procurement of existing and relevant AIDS-related and HFLE curriculum materials from sources inside and outside the country.
- Ensure the local development, production, dissemination of HIV/AIDS and SRH materials and the subsequent use of such materials in education programmes.
- Promote the development of programmes for providing teachers with some skills in psycho-social counselling and stress management.

Information and networking

- Establish and maintain a database on the extent to which HIV/AIDS is impacting on the education system in terms of demand, supply and costs.
- Reform or extend existing Education Management Information Systems (EMIS) to include AIDS-related data that will provide timely information on potential crisis points.

- In co-operation with colleagues in other countries, design and apply a model that will make projections of school enrolments and teacher supply in the circumstances of HIV/AIDS in Caribbean countries.
- In co-operation with the focal points from education ministries in other Caribbean countries, agree on a set of core indicators and critical variables that will allow for regional comparability, and subsequently develop, pilot and apply data-gathering instruments.
- Establish networks within the country and across the Caribbean region for the sharing of information on good practices, programmes addressed to the needs of youth in and out of school, models for responding to orphan needs, HIV/AIDS-in-education statistics, and systemic impacts.

Monitoring, evaluation and research

- Monitor all activities on an ongoing basis.
- Conduct formal periodic evaluations of activities being undertaken and make the necessary adjustments.
- Conduct studies to assess the impact of the disease on institutions,
- Determine how HIV/AIDS is affecting the school participation and performance of the poor, children from poor rural areas; children from densely populated low-cost urban areas, orphans and other vulnerable children.
- Conduct studies to assess the impact of school interventions on the sexual behaviour of young people.
- Develop an HIV/AIDS-oriented research agenda for the education sector (covering such areas as impact assessments at national and local levels; HIV preventive education; teacher preparation in an era of HIV/AIDS; the knowledge and skills young people will need to shape their future in a world with AIDS; the economic impact of HIV/AIDS on the system and its institutions; information needs and utilization; issues of

orphans and vulnerable children; cultural determinants; expressions of sexual identity; violence and sexual abuse).

Orphans and vulnerable children

- Formulate policies to ensure that the education system facilitates orphans and vulnerable children in the exercise of their right to education.
- Ensure that up to the age of 18 orphans and vulnerable children can be assured of educational provision that is completely free.
- Ensure that orphans and children made vulnerable by HIV/AIDS in their families have ready access to such professional psycho-social guidance and counselling as they may need.
- Establish a framework for the provision of active and sustained support for community initiatives that address the educational, emotional and social needs of orphans and vulnerable children.

Planning

- Undertake strategic planning activities and constantly revisit strategic plans to ensure that effective preventive education continues to be delivered throughout the sector and that the sector remains on target in relation to its long-term vision of an AIDS-free society and its medium-term goals for care, support and impact mitigation.
- Translate the strategic plan into realistic and implementable action plans that will specify roles, structures, budgets, quantified and time-bound targets, and milestones.
- Monitor, and where appropriate, provide for the implementation of action plans.
- Design and make use of data-gathering instruments that will provide the detailed information needed to support HIV/AIDS strategic and action planning in the sector.

Policies and procedures

- Develop within the ministry and throughout the sector a common understanding about the nature of the pandemic and its potential impact on education.

- Promote the development of a commonly accepted vision and set of broad strategic principles that will set out the long-term purpose and direction of the sector in its response to HIV/AIDS.

- Facilitate the development of guidelines, regulations and codes of conduct that will interpret policy for educators responsible for implementation.

- Ensure that regulations and procedures pertaining to the safety of learners and educators, ill-health of staff, medical care, access to benefits, and similar matters are reworked so that they allow for circumstances arising from HIV/AIDS.

- Produce and disseminate manuals of procedure for the guidance of education personnel who experience HIV/AIDS-related situations in the course of their duty.

- Ensure that policy statements and regulations consistently adopt a human rights perspective and in particular that they steadily and firmly speak out against gender discrimination, HIV/AIDS-related stigma and discrimination, sexual abuse, and violence in learning institutions.

Publicity

- Disseminate HIV-prevention and AIDS-impact messages through all available channels (print, radio, television, advertisements, electronic).

- Launch and sustain a country-wide publicity campaign on using education to prevent HIV transmission.

- Produce and disseminate newsletters, fliers, information briefs, etc.

- Work with partners to maintain a flow of information/publicity through public and private radio and TV stations, as well as church bulletins, community publications, entertainment events and similar less traditional channels.

- Promote the use of appropriate and culturally relevant publicity or entertainment materials developed in other parts of the world.

School activities

- Promote the active involvement of teachers, NGOs, communities, young people and suitable students, in the delivery of reproductive health, HIV/AIDS and life-skills education within education institutions and for young people who are outside the formal education system.
- Promote the formation of clubs and societies dealing with preventing HIV transmission, tackling substance abuse, providing care and support for the infected, and managing impacts.
- Work with the health sector to ensure that all school personnel have access to user-friendly health services and the necessary supplies.
- Work with other social sectors to ensure that all school personnel have access to voluntary counselling and testing services.

Training for capacity building

- Plan for the training of personnel at all levels, as required by the foregoing; for instance
  - teacher educators, teachers, and peer educators in HIV/AIDS materials, in reproductive health and HIV/AIDS education, in counselling and stress management;
  - administrators and statistical officers in maintaining an AIDS-related management information system;
  - co-ordination officers in developing and maintaining a living matrix of partners/interventions/activities.
- Ensure the establishment of HIV/AIDS-in-the-workplace education programmes for the sector's workforce within the ministry, its branches and institutions.

Youth-friendly health services

- In co-operation with the health sector, develop guidelines on what these will consist of and how they will be provided.
- Encourage local health care centres to set aside special times for the provision of health services to children and young people.
- In collaboration with health personnel, ensure that existing clinics and schools provide the space and time that allow young people confidential access to information, treatment, advice and supplies for conditions related to HIV/AIDS and STIs.
- Provide for trained peer counsellors in secondary and tertiary education institutions who will serve as links between student clients and health care personnel.

Partnerships

Partnerships are crucial to the success of education in confronting HIV/AIDS. No single sector and no agency working in isolation will ever prevail over the epidemic. This can only be accomplished by combining understandings, efforts and resources across the entire public and private sectors and civil society. Both the urgency of the situation and the magnitude of the crisis demand a great willingness to share with others, to participate, plan and work with them, to join in their efforts, and to welcome their participation as partners.

Establishing partnerships at the central level, especially with other government sectors, may be comparatively straightforward. Establishing them at the grassroots level of service delivery, and ensuring that education officials down the line accept the partners on equal and open terms, are the more challenging tasks for education authorities. But they are of the utmost importance in the context of HIV/AIDS since it is at the grassroots level that major action must be taken in relation to prevention and care.

Two major challenges present themselves. One is for those with different backgrounds and affiliations to work together for the common good – ministry officials or school principals working with NGO, community and religious authorities, leaders of faith-based organisations working with one another, and all cooperating harmoniously without animosity, suspicion or a desire to dominate. The role of partners at the grassroots level is to work in harmony with other partners to fight HIV/AIDS, and not to dissipate energies and resources through conflict with one another. The second challenge is to listen. The grassroots and communities are at work. Education officials need to listen and respond to what they hear. Instead of imposing their own priorities, they must see how they can support local initiatives.

Hence, it is crucial that the education ministry maintain strong bonds with other government ministries, NGOs, the private sector, faith-based organisations, the media, and international bodies (above all, regional organisations and those with a Caribbean focus). Recognising that success in the struggle against HIV/AIDS cannot be achieved without multisectoral and multilevel partnerships, the education ministry should strive for vital partnership arrangements involving consolidation of resources, a better definition of respective roles, recognition of the unique contribution coming from each partner, respect for one another, and improved co-ordination. This, in turn, should lead to better focused efforts, all-round improvement in the sense of ownership of activities, more widespread geographical coverage, and more successful implementation of activities.

For an education ministry this would imply:

- establishing a dynamic working relationship with the national AIDS council or programme and its secretariat;
- encouraging or facilitating the active participation of NGOs, FBOs, civic and community leaders, the higher education sub-sector, and all organs of civil society;
- involving teachers, students and community representatives as much as possible as partners in the development, design, and implementation of activities;
- involving parents and communities in curriculum issues;
- encouraging parents and FBOs to communicate with children, from an early age, on issues of sexuality, respect for others as persons, learning to live together peaceably, respecting the human rights of others, gender equity, and HIV prevention;

- making a deliberate effort to ensure the participation of all non-governmental providers of education (private schools, church schools, company schools, etc.);
- working closely with other relevant government ministries, integrating education programmes into theirs where appropriate, and vice versa;
- acknowledging the special role that can be played by universities and other institutions in the higher education sub-sector, especially for the development of new knowledge and understanding;
- bringing the media on board from the outset.

Partnerships with faith-based organisations

Partnerships with faith-based organisations (FBOs) need special attention and encouragement. These organisations are significant providers of AIDS care (*Box 18*). They are well known for their potential to get things done. They play a significant role in the formation of public opinion and the development of attitudes. They have an extensive network of voices at the grassroots level. They reach into every part of a country, and in many cases into every household, in ways that government and civic agencies do not.

Box 18. The provision of AIDS care by a faith-based organisation

Approximately 12 per cent of all AIDS care worldwide is provided by Catholic church organisations, while 13 per cent is provided by Catholic non-governmental organisations. This means that Catholic church-related organisations are providing some 25 per cent of the AIDS care worldwide, making it the largest institution in the world providing direct AIDS care.

Source: Miller, 2001.

The jurisdiction of FBOs and religious authorities 'often includes a number of areas closely connected to HIV/AIDS, such as morality, beliefs about the spiritual bases of disease, and rules of family life and sexual activity,' — areas that other agencies do not deal with. (Liebowitz, 2002: 1). In addition, they have contacts everywhere. Many are in solidarity with worldwide institutions, and their leaders are listened to respectfully and frequently by a wide variety of constituents.

Evidence from countries that have shown some success in controlling HIV infection rates also points to the key role played by FBOs and suggests the need for greater support for major, national-level faith-based initiatives in AIDS prevention. AIDS prevention activities carried out through religious leaders from different faith backgrounds, Christian and Islamic, were significant in preventing the epidemic from spreading more widely in Senegal and in reducing its prevalence in Uganda. Early mobilization of religious leaders and organisations resulted in their active participation in AIDS education and prevention activities. It is noteworthy that in these countries the FBO interventions were focused in the areas of their comparative advantage – partner reduction and the postponement of sexual activity – factors that contributed significantly to success in responding to the epidemic.

Likewise in the Caribbean, FBOs are well placed to make a unique contribution to the struggle with HIV/AIDS. Education ministries should capitalise on this potential by more express efforts to develop good working relationships with these organisations and their leaders. Almost inevitably, this will require care and respect in reaching agreement on curriculum messages that are sometimes contentious, especially those relating to sexuality, condom use and the independence of women. As has been noted already (*Chapter 6*), it is of considerable importance that the partners reach agreement on a common and correct set of messages and that no one of them contradicts, undermines or belittles the messages being communicated by any of the others.

Capacity building

The need for capacity building in the education sector has always been great, but HIV/AIDS has aggravated that need enormously, all the more so in that 'the countries most challenged by EFA and HIV/AIDS objectives are in many cases the ones least equipped to attract resources, use them effectively, and demonstrate their effective use' (World Bank, 2002: 62).

HIV/AIDS affects the need for human capacity in three ways:

1. It increases the scale, scope and urgency of existing tasks, as occurs with efforts to respond to the challenge of orphans and children made vulnerable by the epidemic, or to mobilize the resources needed to support HIV/AIDS interventions.

2. It creates new tasks that call for new skills, as occurs in developing curriculum materials for sexual and reproductive health, or in strategic planning for the education sector in the context of HIV/AIDS.

3. It depletes the human resource base through sickness and death, as occurs with every AIDS-related death of a teacher or education official. In the latter case, capacity is being eroded just at the time when the ministries need all their human resources, and all the wisdom of their institutional memory, to plan for and manage their response to HIV/AIDS. In countries with small populations or fragile education systems, this loss can cause inestimable damage to the entire system, since the individual may be the only available expert in a particular field.

International support for Caribbean initiatives in the fight against HIV/AIDS frequently takes the form of support for capacity building. This is the case with the European Union supported initiative, *Strengthening the Institutional Response to HIV/AIDS/STIs in the Caribbean*, (SIRHASC). The goal of the project is to reduce the spread and impact of the diseases in the Caribbean. It seeks to do this by strengthening regional institutional capacity to plan and coordinate an effective response to the STI/HIV/AIDS epidemics. Two expected outputs, among others, are an increased pool of appropriately skilled personnel able to contribute to effective policy development, planning and implementation of STI/HIV/AIDS programmes, and improved regional capacity to design, implement and evaluate interventions to reduce high-risk behaviour related to the spread of STI/HIV infections.

Education ministries in the region need to do as much for themselves. Denial, insufficient advocacy, lack of awareness, stigma and discrimination may all have contributed to education ministries in the region being as uncertain as those elsewhere in the world in recognising the extent of their responsibility and potential role. But in the meantime, the AIDS situation in the region has grown steadily worse and the need for capacity development to deal with it has grown progressively greater. Education ministries need to strengthen their capacity in the two areas identified by the SIRHASC project. If they are to cope successfully with the tasks they must undertake, the ministries should take steps to:

1.   Increase their pool of appropriately skilled personnel who can contribute to effective policy development, planning and implementation of HIV/AIDS programmes; and

2.   Improve their capacity to design, implement and evaluate interventions to reduce high-risk behaviour related to the spread of HIV infections.

Both short- and long-term measures are needed for this. In the short-term, staff development can be provided through such initiatives as short courses, workshops, intensive short-duration training sessions, or on-the-job support from suitably qualified individuals. But there is also a need for long-term sustained investment in developing the human resources needed to mount an effective response to HIV/AIDS through the education sector. If, as is currently being predicted, the global epidemic will not reach its peak until the second half of the twenty-first century, a long-term sustained investment in ensuring the AIDS competence of education officials would yield rich dividends in equipping ministries for appropriate policy development and implementation. It is said that a child in danger is a child that cannot wait. Education systems are also in danger – in a few instances of being overwhelmed by the epidemic, in the majority of cases of not having the capacity to generate a response. They too cannot wait, but need to direct themselves as a matter of urgency to developing the personnel needed to devise and guide their response.

Strategic planning

Many of the threads that have run through the preceding pages are brought together in the strategic planning process. The process encompasses responding to three straightforward questions:

1. What is the HIV situation in the education sector?

2. What has been done about it so far?

3. What should be done about it in the future? (UNAIDS, 1998a:5)

Strategic planning itself could be defined as a form of planning that has inbuilt provisions for providing a sense of direction in response to changing circumstances. More elaborately, it is a form of planning which secures the appropriate involvement of policy makers, planners, implementers and stakeholders in:

1. The clarification of values and the development of a shared vision.

2. The evaluation of internal and external trends and pressures affecting the organisation or field of activity.

3. The assessment of needs.

4. The identification of desired outcomes.

5. The assignment of priorities to various programmes and initiatives.

6. The specification of activities to achieve these priorities and the time frame within which these activities will be undertaken.

7. The identification of responsible parties to execute these activities, those to whom they will be accountable, and the necessary implementation structures.

8. The broad specification of the human and financial resources needed for the proposed activities and some indication of how these resources will be mobilized.

9. The specification of benchmarks and performance indicators against which progress will be assessed.

10. A continuous process of monitoring and evaluation to adjust to the ever-changing internal and external environment.

A well-developed strategic plan provides guidance to the education sector on how it might change what already exists and move towards a situation where HIV spreads less rapidly, has fewer negative consequences for those infected or affected, and has fewer negative impacts throughout the education system. The approach is led by well-defined goals and objectives, well-developed means to achieve them, preparedness to seize viable opportunities wherever they present themselves, and sensitivity to potential obstacles and hurdles. Important aspects are the reliance on a continuous supply of information about the environment, built-in provisions for providing a sense of direction in response to changing circumstances, and the importance of the process itself. Plan development and implementation are inseparably linked, with focus on the process of plan development as much as on the plan that is developed. This implies that the strategic planning approach relates more to a continuous process than to a planning cycle that may terminate with the production of a plan.

The strategic planning process is key to an education ministry's response to HIV/AIDS. It deals with the real situations that have been uncovered through assessments and analyses. Because it is a continuous process, it continually learns from experience, best practices and non-promising approaches. In addition, being continuous, it is always ready to make provision for the surprising or unexpected features that may accompany the development of the epidemic. Because HIV/AIDS has such long-term effects, the process helps the sector get into a state of readiness so that it can deal with these effects when they come along. It is practical and realistic, with a clear focus on implementation in terms of roles, responsibilities, time-frame, resources and implementation structures. It also establishes a planning culture within an education ministry that can serve it for many years, a feature that is of special importance in the context of the HIV/AIDS epidemic which is projected to persist for a further 50 or more years.

Figure 5 sets out schematically the principal components of the strategic planning process. While most of these have been dealt with already, there are some additional important considerations:

- There is need for wide-ranging participation, to ensure richness, diversity and creativity in plan development and a sense of ownership for plan implementation. The development of a vision that embodies shared values is crucial. Vision refers to a possible and desirable future state of the education sector in its encounter with HIV/AIDS. Values are expressions of how a ministry, concretised in its planning team, thinks things ought to be. They are the criteria against which they will weigh the actions proposed in the plan and that will help to determine priorities. Securing the commitment of ministry personnel and all partners to the vision and implied values is key to all that follows. The vision statement, which does not have to be time-bound, is a dynamic inspirational expression of what the future may look like if the plan to be developed is fully accomplished.

- Goals articulate major accomplishments, within a 3 to 5 year time horizon, which, if attained, would contribute materially to the realization of the vision. Only a limited number of goals should be specified. Objectives define the major achievements that are essential for attaining a goal. There may be several objectives for each goal. Wherever possible, each objective should be Specific, Measurable, Achievable, Realistic and Time-bound (that is, it should be SMART).

- Strategies are steps towards the realisation of objectives. They should indicate the parties responsible for their execution, the lines of accountability, and the time-frame for action. They should also give some indication of the human, financial and other resources needed for action.

Figure 5. The strategic planning process

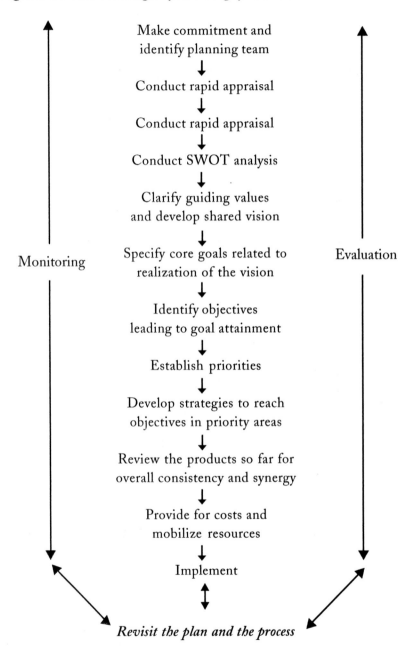

Make commitment and
identify planning team
↓
Conduct rapid appraisal
↓
Conduct rapid appraisal
↓
Conduct SWOT analysis
↓
Clarify guiding values
and develop shared vision
↓
Specify core goals related to
realization of the vision
↓
Identify objectives
leading to goal attainment
↓
Establish priorities
↓
Develop strategies to reach
objectives in priority areas
↓
Review the products so far for
overall consistency and synergy
↓
Provide for costs and
mobilize resources
↓
Implement
↕
Revisit the plan and the process

Monitoring

Evaluation

Source: Adapted from Weindling, 1997; 224.

- There should be benchmarks and performance indicators against which progress would be assessed.

- Progress in implementing the plan should be regularly and systematically assessed, with each item being reviewed and revised in accordance with new information or changed circumstances. This ability to adjust the plan components so that, under changing circumstances, they maintain the sense of direction towards the accomplishment of the vision, is what makes this form of planning strategic.

Resource mobilisation

Education ministries in Caribbean countries that wish to manage the sector proactively in the context of HIV/AIDS need additional human and financial resources. Some of the activities may be supported from national budgets through normal financial and management arrangements. Support for others may come from existing programmes and projects, such as the CARICOM support for HFLE initiatives. But important gaps will remain and these will necessitate the vigorous mobilization of additional support from national, regional and global sources. Resource mobilization for responding to HIV/AIDS should principally aim at increasing the net resources – funds, technical assistance, materials and supplies – available to the education sector to fight the epidemic.

In their efforts to mobilize such resources, education ministries are more likely to be successful if:

- they show evidence of committed and well-informed leadership;
- they have formulated a coherent and comprehensive policy as part of their response to HIV/AIDS; and
- they have developed a realistic and implementable strategic plan to guide the sector's response to the epidemic.

National AIDS Programmes (NAPs) have been established in all territories in the Caribbean. They are responsible for certain policy issues and for the execution of government HIV/AIDS efforts, including the management, planning, and coordination of an expanded national response to HIV/AIDS. The resource mobilization efforts of education ministries stand a greater chance of success when the ministries work in close cooperation with their NAPs or the relevant National AIDS Committee, ensuring that their plans and activities fall within the framework of the guiding principles for the national response and relate to priority areas and strategic goals identified by the national bodies. In some cases, the NAP itself could be the channel through which the ministry receives the necessary additional resources.

Because the epidemic of HIV/AIDS is global, devastating, and security-related, it is a major concern for the United Nations. One result of this is that the United Nations agencies have committed much of their energy, insights and resources to the support of national initiatives to combat the disease. In many areas, they give expression to this through the United Nations Theme Group that meets regularly to consider particular issues relating to relevant national responses. The resource mobilization needs of education ministries could be kept to the fore by extensive interaction with the local UN Theme Group. While the Theme Group would not necessarily be able to provide immediate assistance, it could direct ministries to potential sources or could bring their needs before wider partner organizations.

Education ministries should also be aware of the potential of support from the Global Fund to Fight AIDS, Tuberculosis and Malaria (GFATM) for some of the activities envisaged in their strategic plans for HIV/AIDS and education. Applications to the Global Fund must be developed through Country Coordinating Mechanisms (CCMs), partnerships that include representatives from governments, civil society and persons affected by the diseases. Having to work through CCMs highlights, from another perspective, the importance of wide-ranging partnerships for the education sector, in the design and implementation of its strategic plan for HIV/AIDS and education. A prerequisite for initiatives in this area is that key staff in education ministries be well informed on the Fund and its operations.

Although financial resources are not always immediately available when they are needed or in the amounts needed, combating HIV/AIDS has become such an international priority that programmes embodying an education ministry's strategic response to the epidemic are strongly placed to attract the necessary funding. Although securing the funding may be a problem, often it is not the key problem. The real difficulty lies in the ability to utilize funds effectively and to account for them transparently. Leadership commitment, policy framework, a compelling strategic plan, and strong implementation structures give some assurance that utilization will be efficient and effective. Satisfactory internal financial procedures, applied by qualified staff in a culture of integrity, are the surest guarantee that utilization will be principled and transparent.

Note

1. Readily accessible information on this is provided by the two clearing houses that UNESCO has established.One deals with the impact of HIV/AIDS on education systems, the second with curriculum products and processes relating to HIV prevention education in primary and secondary schools. Details appear in *Appendix 3*.

RESPONDING TO SPECIAL
HIV/AIDS IMPERATIVES

CHAPTER 8

The Special Needs of Orphans and Children Made Vulnerable by HIV/AIDS

The term 'orphan' and the Caribbean social context

HIV/AIDS affects children and young people through orphanhood when parents and guardians die. When planning for care and support for these young people, and others who have lost parents or guardians, it is necessary to understand exactly what is meant by the term 'orphan'. Since the late 1990s, the official definition, as given by UNAIDS and WHO, has become progressively more inclusive. In June 2000, UNAIDS defined an orphan as a child under 15, who had lost either mother or both parents, and it was on this definition that global estimates on AIDS orphans were based (UNAIDS, 2000*b*). A child whose father had died (a paternal orphan) was not included in this definition. Two years later, in July 2002, the definition was extended to include paternal orphans and encompassed any child, aged 0 to 14, who had lost one or both parents. It was on this basis that global estimates of the numbers of orphans living at the end of 2001 were based (UNAIDS, 2002*a*). This same definition was adopted by the *Children on the Brink* Joint Report on Orphan Estimates and Program Strategies (UNAIDS/UNICEF/USAID, 2002).

Since the beginning of 2003, however, in accordance with Article 1 of the Convention on the Rights of the Child,[1] orphan enumerations include all children below the age of 18 who have lost a mother, a father or both parents. This change will clearly mean a revision upwards in published orphan estimates. The new definition is more satisfactory in that it now includes young people between the ages of 15 and 18 who remain dependent on their guardians and whose need for social, economic and psychological support persists after the age of 15. The new extended definition also makes greater allowance for the fact, evidenced from research, that being orphaned means a young person's period of dependency may even be prolonged.

Cultural practices and attitudes towards family and children must also be taken into consideration. One aspect of Caribbean reality is that, in some countries, a large proportion of children are born to unmarried mothers. In many instances the child's father is in a visiting relationship with the mother and he may or may not accept paternal responsibility. In such instances, variable, and often limited, bonding with the biological father occurs. Technically, a child may become a paternal orphan when such a father dies, but this change in status may not be of great significance for the child's emotional status or way of living.

On the other hand, significant bonding tends to occur with members of the extended family, including aunts, uncles and grandparents. Sometimes, the paternal grandparent is the guardian from early in the child's life.

If the biological mother migrates or dies, one or more of these family members will often maintain care of the child and in a few instances may legally adopt the child. In the Caribbean, it is likely that HIV/AIDS would simply be added to the list of reasons why children lose touch with their mothers.

These social arrangements blur, to some extent, the situation of children within a well-defined stable nuclear family. For many couples, the first 'union' status may be the visiting relationship in which the constant for the child is the presence of the mother, who may or may not be living in an extended household with other adults. For some couples, this may be followed by a greater degree of paternal commitment, at which stage the two persons agree to share residence in a common-law union. A significant proportion of these common-law relationships do not eventuate in marriage, but may disintegrate after some years. In the meantime children have been born, children who will move with one or other parent (more commonly the mother) into the life of a single-parent household or new relationship, or who will be absorbed into the family structures of grandparents or other relatives. Many orphans follow a similar route, but the difference for them is that one or both of their parents have died and cannot, therefore, play an active role in their nurturing or upbringing.

The previous chapter drew attention to some of the ways in which HIV/AIDS and violence can interact. These interactions, and the extent of street and home violence, are also relevant to the orphans' situation throughout the Caribbean. Violence is a critical issue for many countries in the region and, as noted already, its scale may dwarf HIV/AIDS in the public consciousness. The fallout affects every person in the community and wider society, engendering fear, agitation and insecurity. Every individual needs the reassurance that all appropriate steps are being taken to tackle this pressing social problem. It would be a cruel irony, however, if confronting violence were to eclipse the challenge posed by the growing number of orphans. The physical, psychological and social development of orphans, just as of others, requires an atmosphere of stability and security. But, more than others, orphans can be at risk of abuse and violence, within the home, on the street, or when in care. The Convention on the Rights of the Child, which has been ratified by every Caribbean country, requires governments to take 'all appropriate legislative, administrative, social and educational measures to protect the child from all forms of physical or mental violence, injury or abuse, neglect or negligent treatment, maltreatment or exploitation' (Article 19). This commitment, which is for every child, is particularly applicable to children who have lost parents or care-givers to HIV/AIDS or other causes.

The scale of the orphans challenge

The most visible demographic impact of the HIV/AIDS epidemic may well be the growth in the number of orphans. *The Children on the Brink 2002* Report estimates that in 88 countries – 41 of them in

Africa, 20 in Asia, 10 in the Caribbean, and 17 in Latin America – the year 2010 will see over 38 million children below the age of 15 who will have lost their mother, father or both parents as a result of AIDS. Many of the paternal orphans (father dead) are likely to lose their mother also within a few years, since if the father, especially the father of a young child, dies as a result of AIDS, the mother will almost certainly be infected also and will not have long to live. The most severely affected countries are likely to be Nigeria, where there may be 3.6 million children below the age of 15 who will have lost one or both parents to AIDS, and Ethiopia where the number is projected to reach just three million (UNAIDS/UNICEF/USAID, 2002).

In the Caribbean, populations are smaller and HIV prevalence rates are lower than in the some of the populous counties of Africa. Nevertheless, because of HIV/AIDS, the region is already experiencing an escalating orphans problem and one that will continue to grow into the future. Detailed estimates are given for 10 Caribbean countries[2] in the *Children on the Brink Report*. For the 10 countries as a group, and in almost all cases for each individual country, the number of orphans due to AIDS and the proportion of children orphaned by AIDS rises steadily across the period 1990-2010 (*Table 5*). Although some decline is projected in the total number of orphans in the period 2001-2010, the proportion of these who will have become orphaned by AIDS will grow larger. The more than tenfold projected increase between 1990 and 2005 in the number of orphans due to AIDS is indicative of the way the epidemic swept through the region in the 1980s and 1990s, causing the premature death of young parents – mostly from 1990 onwards.

Table 5. Orphan estimates for 10 Caribbean countries

Year	Total number of orphans	Total number of orphans due to AIDS	AIDS orphans as percent of all orphans	AIDS orphans as percent of all children
1990	657,000	23,500	3.6	0.2
1995	733,000	128,000	17.5	1.2
2001	792,000	259,000	32.7	2.6
2005	778,000	291,000	37.4	3.0
2010	764000	313,000	41.0	3.2

Source: Derived from *Children on the Brink 2002*, Appendix 1.

Features of the orphans challenge

At the outset, it is important to note that the orphans crisis and orphans challenge are an already existing reality for the Caribbean. As can be deduced from Table 5, it is likely that already in Caribbean countries one in every 40 children under the age of 15 has lost one or both parents to AIDS. The challenge of a large orphaned population is not something that may occur in the future. It is something that is occurring right now and must be addressed in education as in other social sectors.

But although it is occurring right now, in most Caribbean countries the expansion of the AIDS orphan population is likely to be masked for at least two reasons. First, there is a very high proportion of single parent families in the general population of some Caribbean countries because of the union and marriage arrangements already outlined, deaths of spouses from other causes and an increasing rate of divorces. Second, families affected by HIV/AIDS are not always accurately tracked for various reasons, including voluntary seclusion and under-diagnosis.

In so far as it is due to HIV/AIDS, the orphans problem does not necessarily have to become larger. Its growth could be stemmed by ensuring that every HIV infected parent has access to the antiretroviral therapy and drugs needed to keep him or her alive. This calls for immediate action, since it is individuals who are already HIV infected who are likely to contribute to growth in the number of orphans.

However, if for any reason these infected parents do not get access to optimal care, including antiretroviral therapy, it is inevitable that the problem will continue to grow. The projections in *Table 5* show that in the Caribbean such growth in orphan numbers could reach the stage in 2010 when approximately one in every 30 children under the age of 15 would have lost one or both parents to the epidemic.

Second, it must always be borne in mind that, no more than any others infected or affected by HIV/AIDS, orphans are not statistics. They are flesh and blood human beings. They are children who have been cheated by life. Almost all of them are struggling to live without that one feature which gives meaning to a young life and which no social welfare or agency programme can provide – the love of a connected and concerned parent.

Third, the orphans are young. UNICEF data show that around half the orphans in sub-Saharan Africa are aged ten or below – 30 per cent are aged between 6 and 10, 18 per cent are under the age of five, while the mean age of orphaning is 6.2 years (Mugabe, Stirling and Whiteside, 2002). There is no reason to think that it would be any different in Caribbean countries.

Fourth, if one parent has died of AIDS, the likelihood is quite high that the other parent will be HIV positive and will die of the disease. This means that children who have lost one parent to the disease are quite likely to experience the loss of the second parent also. This is because if one partner is infected, then in most cases the other will already also be HIV-infected. The child will therefore almost certainly have to undergo the trauma of being orphaned a second time, and this sooner rather than later.

A further critical feature of orphanhood is that it is an enduring state or condition that lasts throughout the years of a child's life and accompanies the child into adulthood. A six year-old orphaned child will need support, care and protection for at least another ten or 12 years. A two year-old orphaned child will need almost a generation of care. In this, the orphans crisis differs from other problems of development. If there is a water shortage in an area, it can usually be addressed by the one-off event of extending the water network or sinking a well and thereafter giving periodic attention to maintenance.

One-off interventions and periodic attention are totally inadequate for orphans. Instead, they need sustained regular support and attention over a decade or more. Responding to their needs demands more than the short-term perspective of five-year plans. It requires sustained commitment that will remain faithful to individual orphans for as long as is needed, seeing one wave after another of fragile, vulnerable young people through to maturity and adulthood.

One other important aspect of the HIV/AIDS situation in relation to children is that while it is frequently possible to identify the orphaned child, there may be hundreds of other children affected by the epidemic who cannot be identified so readily but who suffer from its myriad impacts. Orphans are the tip of the iceberg. Theirs are the visible faces that draw attention to the countless other children in an AIDS affected society, who may differ from orphans only in that their parents have not yet died, but who experience the poverty, stigma, uncertainty, and hopelessness that so frequently accompany AIDS in a household or community.

Consequences of HIV/AIDS for children

Very correctly, society throughout the region pays a great deal of attention to meeting the basic needs of children for food, clothing, accommodation, health care, and education. In Caribbean countries, social services for orphaned or abandoned children are generally good, though caregivers may not always know what is available or may be reluctant to access services because they fear that by doing so they would become identified as individuals who were somehow 'associated' with HIV/AIDS.

But in general, society pays much less attention to meeting the needs of orphans or vulnerable children for love, affection and security. These are not commodities that can be accumulated over time or provided through welfare arrangements. An important book by two economists has asked a telling question about the 'cost of a cuddle forgone' (Barnett and Whiteside, 2002: 7). This is one of a host of human problems, with no quantifiable or economic dimensions, that HIV/AIDS raises and that society is only beginning to be dimly aware of. The World Summit on Sustainable Development, held in Johannesburg in September 2002, alerted the world to the fact that development cannot be sustained without care for the environment. But even more fundamentally, the human development of children cannot be sustained without an environment of love and security, and it is precisely these that HIV/AIDS places under threat.

The threat begins long before the finality of death eventuates. HIV is a slow-working virus that may spend ten or more years working on the body's immune system before it has weakened it sufficiently for life-threatening opportunistic illnesses to take hold. When they do, they may course through the body with an inhuman and devastating savagery. As with others in the household, the children experience the daily trauma of seeing mother or father enduring the devastating effects and remorseless suffering of AIDS and its culmination in what is often a dehumanizing death (*Box 19*).

Box 19. Becoming an orphan

Becoming an orphan of the epidemic is rarely a sudden switch in roles. It is slow and painful, and the slowness and pain have to do not only with loss of a parent but also with the long-term care which that parent's failing health may require.... A young girl of eight or nine may be used to caring for younger siblings: she is unprepared to care for her mother, father, or both of them.... Coping with a parent who is weak and requires food to be cooked or water to be brought is one thing. Coping with a parent's severe diarrhoea, declining mental function and mood changes is quite another (Barnett and Whiteside, 2002: 206).

In addition to the emotional distress arising from circumstances such as these, children whose parents have died from AIDS suffer numerous adverse social consequences:

- They may arouse sentiments of fear and suspicion in others; are likely to experience stigmatization and discrimination; and are often the subjects of cruel jests, taunts and unreasonable demands.

- They are more likely than non-orphans to be malnourished and under-weight.

- Although the evidence is mixed, in general orphans are more likely than non-orphans to be out of school (Ainsworth and Filmer, 2002. See also below).

- The proportion of children aged 5 to 14 who work more than 40 hours a week is higher among orphans than non-orphans (Mugabe *et al.*, 2002: 3).

- A large proportion of orphans end up as street children.

- Emotional vulnerability and financial desperation expose orphans to greater risk of sexual abuse and exploitation.

- Their vulnerability to sexual abuse puts orphans at a higher risk than other children of becoming HIV infected.

Orphan care

It is critically important that orphaned children are allowed to develop in an atmosphere that is normal and emotionally secure. This has two very practical implications for policy and practice. One is that orphans should not be singled out as a special category. Above all, those whose parents have died from AIDS should not be categorized as 'AIDS orphans'. Labelling them in this way can increase stigmatization, discrimination and harm for these children. Such labelling is all the more undesirable in situations where there are also large numbers of other vulnerable children whose parents are still alive. Within communities, assistance should be directed to the most vulnerable children and households, regardless of orphan status, and one can generally rely on communities to identify those who are in greatest need and most vulnerable.

The second practical recommendation relates to the importance of school education for orphaned children. School attendance is one of the greatest antidotes to an orphan's sense of loss, insecurity and uneasiness. Schooling is strongly characterised by normality and routine, factors that help everybody, children included, make sense of disturbing and bewildering situations. It provides a social milieu where the orphaned child can relate to peers and adults in situations of ordinariness, rationality and regularity. In this way it helps the child develop a renewed sense of efficacy in relation to life and its happenings, restores some of the lost confidence, and offers hope that life can go ahead. 'School restores structure to young lives; it provides a measure of stability in the midst of chaos; it trains the mind, rehabilitates the spirit, and offers critical, life-sustaining hope to a child in the face of an otherwise uncertain future' (Donovan, 2000: 3).

In the Caribbean, there may be need for special measures to ensure school participation and performance on the part of male orphans. This is because, unlike other parts of the world, the region experiences a gender disparity that is more favourable to girls than to boys, in terms of numbers, life expectancy in school, and school performance. Data for orphans is very sparse, but the little that is available shows that their situation is similar to that of the general population of children in Caribbean countries – enrolment ratios are higher for female than for male orphans (Ainsworth and Filmer, 2002, *Table 7*).

A fundamental guiding principle for the care of orphans is that, following the death of one or both parents, they remain within their communities in a family-like setting with an adult guardian or caregiver. This is often accomplished through the extended family: the orphans remain with or are incorporated into a family with which they have blood ties. Ideally, they should also stay with their own sibling group and live in the familiar surroundings of a known community. They should also be party to decisions affecting them and should not be treated either as statistics or virtually as chattels to be disposed of.

Household arrangements for responding to an orphan's needs

Any of three different household arrangements can be made when responding to the needs of orphans, abandoned children or children whose vulnerability is accentuated by HIV/AIDS. They can be shown how to fend for themselves in child or sibling-headed households; placed in institutional care; or integrated into a functioning household. The least satisfactory arrangement is the child or sibling-headed household. In such a household, the children place themselves under the guidance of one of their number, usually the oldest, who by unspoken consent assumes economic and quasi-parenting responsibilities for the others. Generally those in one group will be siblings or at least have close ties with one another, though similar households are also formed by street-children whose bond is their common need for survival. Sibling households, where the household head may be in the late teens, frequently establish themselves because brothers and sisters who have lived and worked together in caring for their sick and dying parents want to preserve their sense of identity, worth and dignity by remaining together.

Households headed by minors are less common in the Caribbean than in Africa, but there is growing evidence that they are coming into being, sometimes because of the migration abroad of parents and sometimes because of the death of parents. A child/sibling-headed household is far from being an ideal way of providing for the care needs of orphans and vulnerable children. Access to basic food, health, education and social needs is on a very precarious footing for children in such households. The possibility of school attendance may be precluded by the need for everybody in the household, including even the youngest, to work to generate the resources needed for survival. Nevertheless, even in such households, anecdotal evidence speaks of older children who are sensitive to the importance of education for their younger siblings and who make heroic efforts to ensure that at least some of them attend school.

Children who are completely bereft of adult family members or who have been remanded for 'bad behaviour' are often accommodated in 'children's homes', orphanages or 'places of safety', as they are called in some Caribbean countries. At the time of writing, no public authority was known that had made special provision for children from families experiencing HIV or AIDS. In a few instances, however, private and religious organisations had begun to accommodate HIV-positive children in orphanages dedicated to this purpose.

Although it has some place, institutional care for the large number of children being orphaned or otherwise rendered vulnerable by HIV/AIDS is less practical on grounds of cost and capacity and less desirable in social terms than providing a comparable level of care with a family or community. Institutional care is several times more costly than community care. Moreover, the needs that the AIDS epidemic is creating greatly exceed the capacity of institutions. Further, institutional care is not a desirable way of meeting the needs of orphans and vulnerable children because institutions do not respond well to the developmental and long-term needs of children. One result is that children who have lived for many years in orphanages often find it difficult to adjust to the social and economic situations they encounter when they leave these institutions (Jackson, 2002: 285-291). It has also been well established that the incidence of cross-infection is higher in institutions than in community or family homes and this may be of dire consequence for orphans, some of whom may themselves be HIV-positive.

In addition to the risks already mentioned, there is also the danger that orphanages may be viewed as a way of escape – for the child from poverty and for the relatives from responsibility. A further hazard is a development that is being experienced in parts of Africa and from which Caribbean countries may not be immune – namely, the phenomenon of 'orphan farms' where developers provide institutional homes for children in the expectation of considerable government and donor support, but with only a small part of this going to the benefit of the orphans (Barnett and Whiteside, 2002).

Nevertheless, orphanages have a place as a temporary arrangement while negotiations are under way for the within family placement of an orphan. They also have a place as a home for abandoned children, especially those who are HIV-positive, and for children in especially difficult circumstances, such as post-conflict situations, and 'problem' children who cannot be placed in a family.

The most satisfactory response to orphan needs is placement within a family, preferably with relatives who form part of the extended family. The outcomes are likely to be satisfactory to all concerned when the family in question willingly agrees to integrate orphaned relatives and has the financial and other resources needed to do so. But if the family is reluctant, or does not have or receive the financial resources to cater for the additional members, the outcomes can be tragic. In such households, orphans may sense that they are unwelcome; they may experience discrimination and abuse (verbal, physical and sexual) or be stigmatised because their parents died from AIDS. They may not receive the support they need to enable them to attend school regularly and profitably, and may be required to undertake an excessive amount of household work.

Where households are already poor, the incorporation of orphans may drive them further into poverty as they strive to provide food, clothing and a home for a larger number, but with no commensurate increase in income. They may give the impression that they are managing, but in reality they may be coping neither with poverty nor with orphan care.

The education of orphans

Although the situation varies between and within countries, the bulk of the evidence shows some differences in school attendance rates between orphans and non-orphans, particularly in those coming from lower income families. A striking example is Haiti where the enrolment difference between children with both parents dead and those with both parents living is very pronounced. In this case the difference is much greater in the poorer, rather than in the wealthier section of the population (*Table 6*). Reports from child welfare professionals in other Caribbean countries also speak of orphans, whom family arrangements have placed on an informal basis with relatives from the extended family, attending school quite irregularly or even not attending at all if pressures on household finances are experienced. It seems that there is less likelihood of this happening when there are formal fostering arrangements that involve government child support grants – these may include provision for special educational expenses, such as fees where these are needed, textbooks or examinations costs – and some supervision by child welfare officials to ensure that the fostered child is being properly looked after and has access to the necessary medical and educational services.

Table 6. School enrolment of children aged 7-14 by orphan status and household wealth, Haiti, 1994-1995

Orphan Status	Percentage enrolled in school		
	All Children	Children from the poorest 40%	Children from the richest 20 %
Not orphaned (both parents still living)	77	66	92
Orphaned (both parents dead	60	44	76

Source: Ainsworth and Filmer, 2002, Appendix 4.

Much of the concern and care for orphans tends to be directed to younger children. This is reflected even in the international data provided by UNAIDS, with orphan enumerations up to the end of 2002 including only those aged 0 to 14 years. The more recent decision to extend the definition of an orphan to include children below the age of 18 who have lost one or both parents is important in directing attention to the needs of teenagers who are orphans. These may not be able to meet the costs sometimes associated with education and training programmes for young people. Because of their age, they may not benefit from social welfare arrangements. As a result, the households where they live may need special financial assistance to ensure their participation in relevant programmes. In some cases, also, these teenage orphans will need special psychological support and counselling, particularly if during the early, transitional years of their adolescence, their parents died from AIDS-related causes.

Issues related to the education and training of orphaned children and youth to which educational personnel in Caribbean countries should give attention include:

- Working with a wide range of partners to identify those in the community or catchment area who have been orphaned, because of AIDS or any other cause, so that the scale of the challenge arising from orphaned children and youth is well understood and built into financial and other planning.

- Playing an active part in ensuring that all children and youth are either in school or in an appropriate education or training programme, and are receiving quality education.

- Ensuring that the necessary financial support exists so that no orphaned child or youth is prevented from participation in a relevant education or training programme of good quality by inability to pay or to meet the costs of examinations, uniforms, educational materials, or other education-related needs.

- Paying particular attention to the school and education needs of orphaned girls, since these are frequently required to assume a disproportionate share of the responsibilities associated with caring for siblings and parents who are ill.

- Establishing that throughout the education sector and in every one of its institutions, public and private, the prevailing atmosphere is one of acceptance and welcome for orphaned children and youth, without any trace of uneasiness, stigma or discrimination because their parents have died from AIDS. The practical manifestation of this is zero tolerance for any expression of stigma or discrimination, irrespective of the source.

- Supporting community innovations that seek to respond in creative and innovative ways to the education and training needs of orphaned and disadvantaged children and youth.

- Establishing counselling services and training programmes in psycho-social counselling that will provide the psychological support frequently needed by orphans and other vulnerable children who have been affected by HIV/AIDS in their families. Concretely, this may necessitate training workshops and training programmes for teachers and other education personnel, as well as modifications to include more extensive coverage of child counselling in pre-service teacher preparation programmes.

• Placing orphanhood, the strengthening of family, community caring and coping capacity, and managing HIV/AIDS trauma high on the research agenda in universities and social research units. The majority of the children who have been orphaned and otherwise made vulnerable by AIDS are living within their extended families and communities, but scientific understanding is limited on how families/communities actually cope, the psychological, material and financial problems they experience, and where there is potential danger of breakdown.

Some further observations should be noted in relation to responding to the orphans challenge. There is perhaps a greater need here for a dynamic coalition of all partners. Educational responses cannot be separated from those in the wider social sphere. Education personnel must remain aware of and learn from the coping strategies devised by families, communities and other agencies. The education sector must be deeply involved in responding to the orphans challenge, but it cannot do so all on its own. Its response must be developed in collaborative involvement with other central and local government institutions, NGOs, faith-based organisations, and communities.

Second, dealing with orphans and other children made vulnerable by HIV/AIDS requires a bottom-up approach. Very rightly, the majority of orphans live in communities and for the greater part are supported by community-based initiatives. The various partners, including the education sector, should promote and support such initiatives. These must, however, remain initiatives of the community, developed at the local level and not in central or local government offices, and not even in the offices of NGOs or faith-based organisations. A guiding principle for agencies that are external to families and communities — including the education sector — is that they should seek to strengthen the capacity of families and communities to care for their orphaned children. They should never seek to supplant them.

Finally, it is important that education and other areas recognise the silent and almost invisible growth in the magnitude and geographic extent of the orphans challenge. The challenge is escalating day by day and there is need to plan and take action quickly before the dimensions of the problem grow so large that they become unmanageable. In many societies, AIDS has become virtually unmanageable. Steps should be taken to ensure that nothing similar happens with orphans. This is a special challenge not only for education ministries but also for universities, colleges of education, individual schools, and training establishments and programmes. Collectively they must devise an adequate educational response to ensure that in imaginative and creative ways children and youth orphaned as a result of AIDS or other occurrence can be educated in a way that will help to compensate them for their human loss while preparing them for a full and satisfying human life.

One final and almost unanswerable question must be raised about orphans and how the education system can respond to their needs. The basic problem is not of getting them into schools or educational programmes. The crucial problem is not even ensuring their survival within extended families and communities. The fundamental issue is the kind of adult they will grow up to be. An enormous number would have been cheated of their childhood. From a very early age they would have been 'juvenile adults'. They would have been catapulted from infancy or very early childhood into adult status with responsibilities without passing through the formative years of a normal childhood. They would not have known the love, security and stability within which the human personality normally develops. Some would have known little more than the company of a very much older generation, some only the company of inexperienced children like themselves. Some would have moved from one surrogate parent to another. Some would have been almost forcibly separated from the only stable focus they had known in their lives – their own siblings and the familiar surroundings of the place where they were reared.

Can the education they receive compensate for this absence of normal human upbringing? Can it help to ensure that when they pass to full adult status these 'juvenile adults' will do so as mature individuals, capable of founding and sustaining a family? HIV/AIDS and the resultant orphans crisis are too recent an experience for these questions to be answered with any certainty. But perhaps the questions point to the need to ensure that all educational programmes endeavour to compensate orphans for much that they have lost in life, that they provide them with security, stability, affection, human warmth, and an opportunity for joy, gaiety and laughter.

Notes

1.   'For the purposes of the present Convention, a child means every human being below the age of 18 years unless, under the law applicable to the child, majority is attained earlier' (CRC, Article 1). With the exception of two states, neither of them in the Caribbean, this Convention has been ratified by every state in the world.

2.   Bahamas, Barbados, Belize, Cuba, Dominican Republic, Guyana, Haiti, Jamaica, Suriname, and Trinidad and Tobago.

CHAPTER 9

Reaching Young People Outside the Formal Education System

There are several reasons why it is necessary to pay special attention to HIV prevention for young people who are outside the formal education system:

1. They form a large part of the population. More than half of the overall Caribbean population is under the age of 24, with roughly 33 per cent under the age of 15 and another 20 per cent between 15 and 24. A large proportion of the latter group does not participate in any formal education programme. In Jamaica, a rapid drop in school enrolment after the age of 14 resulted in 22 per cent of the 12 -18 year-olds being out of school in 1998, while less than 21 per cent of 17-18 year olds from the poorest quintile are enrolled in formal education programmes (Williams, 2002: 236).

2. They are at the centre of the epidemic. Young people are at the heart of the HIV/AIDS epidemic, globally and regionally. Globally, an estimated 11.8 million young people aged 15 -24 are living with HIV/AIDS. Moreover, about half of all new adult infections – about 6,000 each day – are occurring among young people in this age group. In the Caribbean, 50 per cent of AIDS cases are diagnosed in the 25 -34 age group. Because of the time it takes to progress from HIV infection to a fully diagnosed AIDS case, this actually means that many of these individuals became infected when they were in their teens or

early twenties (CRSPAH, 2000: 9). Although data from several countries are incomplete, indications are that a significant proportion of these young people were outside of the formal educational system when they became infected.

3.   They are the AIDS generation. Today's young people have never known a world without HIV/AIDS. Their generation carries a heavier burden of HIV infection than any previous generation of young people and has the potential to transmit this infection to the next generation. Significant numbers among them are HIV infected but are not aware of that fact. Because the epidemic among them remains largely invisible, to the young people themselves and to society as a whole, they are in danger of underestimating it as a somewhat troubling reality that one can learn to live with. Their own protection and the protection of future generations necessitate comprehensive attention to their HIV education and prevention needs.

4.   They lack information. Young people's vulnerability to infection is aggravated by insufficient knowledge on how HIV/AIDS can be prevented. Surveys have found that in Suriname only 27 per cent of 15-24 year-old young women had sufficient knowledge to protect themselves from HIV infection and in Trinidad and Tobago only 33 per cent (UNICEF, 2002, *Table 8*). In Haiti, 32 per cent of young women do not know that healthy-looking people can be infected with HIV.

5.   They are strongly influenced by the stigma and prejudice manifested throughout society. Stigma, silence and shame make it difficult for young people to adopt HIV prevention strategies, seek HIV or STI testing, adhere to treatment, or disclose their HIV status to sexual partners. The fact that they share these negative attitudes to HIV with the wider society makes it even more necessary to support them with programmes that will bring these issues out into the open. The extent of the fear and prejudice against those with HIV/AIDS can be gauged from responses to questionnaires in Cuba and the Dominican

Republic, where only 25 per cent of young women aged 15 to 24 said they would buy food from an HIV-positive shopkeeper, or thought that a teacher who is HIV-positive but looks healthy should be allowed to continue to work, (*Figure 6*). The fear and prejudice seem to be even greater in Suriname and Trinidad and Tobago. All young people need help in overcoming these prejudices, which, as *Figure 5* shows, are also shared by those older than them.

Figure 6. Percentage of young women expressing a positive attitude towards people living with HIV/AIDS

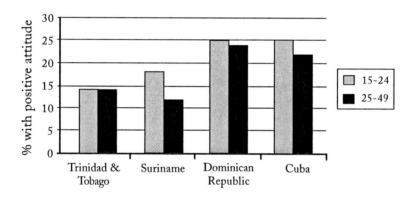

Source: UNAIDS/UNICEF/WHO, 2002: 25.

6. Girls are at special risk. In the majority of Caribbean countries, HIV prevalence rates among young women are higher than those among young men (*Table 4*). Young women run high risks of infection because a) their partners are often older men who are more likely to be HIV infected, and b) because of the 'hidden story of coercive sex, rape, incest, domestic violence, and predatory 'sugar daddies' that young girls must cope with' (CRSPAH, 2000: 9). Young women who do not participate in formal education programmes need approaches that will equip them with correct knowledge, improve their negotiating skills, and familiarise them with the range of available services.

7. Their needs are not adequately catered for. Large-scale HIVprevention programmes are difficult to access and few are directed towards young people without some institutional base in education. To the extent that they are catered for at all, their needs tend to be met by programmes that are small in scale and seldom co-ordinated or harmonised with one another.

8. Young people outside of the education system, and those within, are a force for positive change. They are the region's greatest hope against the epidemic. Where they have been able to access appropriate knowledge, skills and means, they have shown that they are capable of adopting risk-free behaviour. In countries where the tide has turned against HIV/AIDS, or is beginning to turn, the change has come about primarily because young people have been given the information, tools and incentives they need to make responsible and life-affirming choices. Being still at a learning stage, young people can adopt new practices more easily than adults and often prove more dynamic than adults in contributing to HIV prevention, care and support, and impact mitigation.

9. The world has made commitments on their behalf. Through the United Nations Declaration of Commitment, the world has manifested special interest in those between the ages of 15 and 24, most of whom do not take part in any formal educational programme. The world commitment is to ensure that by 2010 HIV prevalence among young men and women aged 15 to 24 will be reduced by 25 per cent and that by the same year 95 per cent of these young people will have access to the information, education and services they need to reduce their vulnerability to HIV infection (UNGASS, 2001: §47, 53). In the absence of a strong commitment to programmes for young people outside the formal education system, there can be no hope of achieving these targets.

Addressing the need

The major issues that arise in programming for the HIV preventive education needs of young people who are not in schools or third level programmes are:

- How to market the programme to ensure that the target audience is reached.
- How to achieve universal coverage.
- Who should be responsible for delivering the programme.
- What the programme should deal with.
- How it should be structured.
- What learning methods should be used.
- How the programme should be evaluated.

The focus of an HIV prevention education programme for young people not attending education institutions is on the range of strategies on youth. Basically, the programme should deal with issues that are appropriate to the needs and interests of young people in an HIV/AIDS-affected environment (*Box 20*). Hence it should respond to the need for accurate and scientific information about the disease itself, how it is transmitted and the protection measures that can be adopted. It should address young people's reproductive and sexual health needs frankly and constructively. It should seek to equip participants with the skills, including the life skills, which will enable them to put knowledge into practice. In all of this, the programme would not differ in basic content from the HIV/AIDS, sexual and reproductive health, and life skills elements in the school curriculum (*Chapter 6*). There would however be very considerable differences in the methodology and setting of the communication process and in the necessary back-up services. In the context of the existing and emerging sexual patterns in the Caribbean, successful HIV prevention programmes for young people would also need to challenge the prevalent ideologies and stereotypes of masculinity and femininity that champion an assertive, sexually domineering, free-ranging multiple-partner image for men and boys, and a submissive, yielding, loyal partner image for women and girls.

Box 20. The voices of youth

In June 2002, UNESCO's International Bureau of Education published a special issue of *Prospects* devoted to Education for HIV/ AIDS Prevention. Recognising the importance of the active involvement of young people in developing interventions and (in some cases) implementing them, the issue included statements from young people from around the world.

From St. Kitts and Nevis

'Education about the epidemic should be more appropriate to the needs and interests of the youth of the world. Our attention needs to be captured and held in a way that will make us more alert to the real crisis that threatens us and more responsible about our personal and social behaviour' (Eustace T. Wallace, male, aged 18).

From the Russian Federation

'Now, I always think about healthy ways of life, about my future and I try to protect my friends from 'unknown' relationships. This virus can infect any of us. That is why we need to be serious about our sexual behaviour, thinking about our future and about our kids' (Anna Shektman, female, aged 20).

From Israel

'I was 19 years old when I first learned I was HIV positive.... It came as a total shock. I had heard about AIDS before. It was even mentioned once in sex education classes at school. But for me that was 'other people's disease'. I knew about Rock Hudson; I knew that Freddy Mercury died of AIDS. I felt immune ... I thought you can distinguish who is HIV infected and who is not by just looking at them. My boyfriend looked OK. But he was infected, and we did not know that. Looking back, I was dumb. And I was also not so ready for sexual life. I couldn't negotiate.... I was also very sure it would never happen to me' (Inbal Gur Arieh, female, aged 24).

The structuring and delivery of interventions refer to three areas that are important in all settings, but are critical when dealing with young people who do not attend education institutions. The first is to engage the young people themselves, promoting their active participation as communicators and learners. Involving young people in prevention efforts educates them about HIV and increases their sense of responsibility. Involving the target audience in programme planning helps to ensure that interventions are appropriate and respond to audience needs. In particular, peer to peer (youth to youth) programmes deserve to be encouraged. Many strategies for youth education now rely heavily on this approach. Teenagers and those in their early twenties, even those in high-risk groups, can be very effective educators for HIV prevention. Apart altogether from the formal or informal settings of HIV prevention programmes, many young people turn to their peers for information and advice on sexual matters. Peer education seeks to capitalize on this ease of sharing.

For this approach to be effective, adults need to begin the process by training the peer educators to ensure that they have correct knowledge, that the educators have themselves acquired the skills they will demonstrate, and that the educators are adept at using basic communication techniques. In the successful peer education programme used by the Red Cross in parts of the Caribbean, adults have continued to make themselves available as advisors to the active peer educators even after the initial training period was over.

The other two areas that need attention are the availability of youth-friendly health services and the promotion of voluntary and confidential HIV counselling and testing (VCT). Ideally, youth-friendly health services 'provide a full range of services and information to young people and are welcoming, confidential, conveniently located and affordable. The staff members do not patronize or lecture young people and give them plenty of time to talk' (UNAIDS/UNICEF/WHO, 2002: 30). The importance of VCT cannot be overstressed. For those who test negative, there is an incentive to remain so. For those who test positive, there is greater chance that they will receive the care and treatment that will help them to live a full and positive life. It may not always be possible for these two sets of services to be an integral part of every outreach programme to youth. But, once such services become available in each country, it should become the norm for every programme to direct its participants to them.

Partners and participants

'Knowledge, education and skills are key words in education for HIV/ AIDS prevention. In many countries affected by HIV/AIDS these are being provided in separate and isolated 'projects'. Although this phase is extremely necessary and important, this approach might not be sufficiently useful in the long-term effort to influence the attitudes and behaviours of young people' (Braslavsky, 2002: 4). In their original context these words referred to the in-school mainstreaming of HIV preventive education. But they also capture what is a major problem in the provision of such education for young people outside of the formal education system. Proposals abound on the strategic principles that should be adopted for addressing this problem. There is much less guidance on developing these principles into action plans in ways that will ensure co-ordination and harmonisation, will avoid fragmentation, duplication, overlap and the neglect of various groups, and yet will ensure that scope is left for the vitality and variety of cooperating partners. The needs are almost conflicting: how to involve all partners, their strengths and interests, but simultaneously how to avoid excessive 'projectisation'.

When the response to HIV/AIDS or any other important issue is mainly through externally funded projects, there is uncertainty about the locus of control, roles and responsibilities. This seems to apply in the area of preventive HIV education for young people outside the formal education system in many parts of the world, including the Caribbean. At present, in projects for 'out-of-school' youth:

- the depth, duration, and coverage of partners' and agencies' responses vary considerably;
- there is a lack of comprehensive knowledge as to what is happening;

- there is a lack of the co-ordination needed to ensure the widest possible coverage and that no groups are overlooked;
- information-sharing and networking appear to be at a minimum.

But the compactness of the communities within the Caribbean, and the size of many of the territories, should make it possible to remedy this situation. If the Caribbean could bring this about and eventually come forward with well-co-ordinated national and regional strategies and action plans for bringing HIV preventive education to every young person not attending an educational institution, it would be making excellent use of the comparative advantage afforded by relatively small tight-knit populations and communities in dynamic contact with one another. The world would stand to gain enormously and to learn much from such a development in the region.

In many territories in the region, the ministry responsible for education also has responsibility for youth affairs and sometimes also for one or more of sports, culture, welfare or development. This unification of responsibilities within a single ministry provides a strong basis for a unified approach to meeting the HIV prevention education needs of all young people, regardless of their ongoing educational status. Where a ministry's formal responsibility does not extend beyond education, it can help if it defines for itself the limits of its responsibilities – the age group where its responsibility starts and the age or educational group where its responsibility ends – and then ensure that within those limits the necessary HIV prevention education is made available. Thus, some countries have stated clearly that the responsibility of the education ministry extends to all young people between the ages of three and 16, whether or not they formally attend educational institutions.

This exercise in self-definition can reveal areas or groups for whom the ministry is not providing educational services, including HIV preventive education. Children who live on the street are an obvious example. In some circumstances, orphans may be another category of neglected children. But there can be other groups, especially among the older age cohorts where many young people leave school before the statutory age. These are ones with whom the ministry should be specially concerned.

In addition, almost every ministry whose exclusive remit is education has a structure for attending to continuing or lifelong education. Working in close collaboration with their National AIDS Programmes, social sector ministries, and private and community organisations, ministries could use the services of such units to bring about more focused efforts to reach overlooked groups.

In every effort to make HIV prevention education services available to young people outside the formal education system, there are essentially two players – the target group and the providing group. The challenge is to mobilise both of these so that they come together in some organised way to deal with the area of HIV preventive education. At the level of the target group, the major problem may be lack of interest or demand. At the level of the provider, the major problem may be supplying the necessary educational services in a consistent, coordinated, reliable and accurate way.

Stimulating interest and demand on the part of young people in the various situations in which they find themselves – at work; unemployed; living in ghetto situations; living in hard-to-access rural districts; comparatively well-off; living in poverty and possibly even in destitution; living on the street – can be very challenging. The education sector should do what it can through its institutions to speak to such groups, but mostly its work in this area will be through the support it provides for social workers and others who are more directly involved. What is crucial is that the sector is seen to provide such support, thereby demonstrating that it sees itself as sharing in the responsibility of bringing HIV prevention education to every young person — whether or not they are attending education institutions.

But the education sector can play an even more substantial role in the provision of education programmes for those who are not attending its institutions. For the greater part it will do this in partnership with a variety of government, business and social actors. Among the latter, community-based organisations, faith-based organisations and churches are of special importance because of the way they reach into the hearts of communities. An education ministry commands substantial human and physical resources, access to which would facilitate other ministries, the private sector, NGOs, faith-based organisations and others in setting up HIV programmes for young people. In the crisis situation that HIV/AIDS represents, school premises could be made available to organisations providing HIV programmes for young people, at times when they are not in use for regular institutional programmes. Teachers and other education personnel, who have knowledge and skills that could be deployed in HIV programmes for out-of-school youth, could be encouraged to participate in curriculum development and delivery of such programmes. Ministries could show their support for such participation by recognizing it as part of a member of staff's workload or as grounds for promotion and career advancement.

In these and similar ways, education ministries can demonstrate the importance they attach to ensuring that ways are found for addressing the HIV prevention education needs of young people who are outside of its formal education structures.

Finally, the education sector can draw on its expertise to fill the many gaps in information about programmes for young people. The Caribbean, in common with other regions in the world, has seen the development of a large number of programmes that target young people on HIV/AIDS and reproductive health matters. Many of the programmes have been developed by NGOs, FBOs and other community organisations. Some target those who are attending school. Others are directed towards out-of-school youth. Still others work across all categories of young people, within or outside the formal education system. These programmes vary considerably in coverage, duration and content. But despite their number and variety, information about them is very sparse. There is little information on good practice or programme effectiveness, and hence little potential for learning from one another.

Education ministries could participate in filling this information gap. Working with partners at both national and regional levels, they could address the problem in two ways:

1. By developing, disseminating and maintaining an annotated directory of current and recent HIV prevention programmes targeted at young people in their countries (or across the Caribbean); and

2. By developing and disseminating a handbook of case studies. This would give detailed information on a selected number of these programmes, with a focus on promising programmes or those that seem to be effective in meeting the UNGASS objective of ensuring that all young people have access to the information, education and services they need to reduce their vulnerability to HIV infection.

The availability of these resources would provide programme managers with information on what has been tried elsewhere and would support them in developing interventions that respond more clearly to the needs of their target audiences. The information would also help in directing young people to programmes that would respond to their needs, in identifying areas and groups who are not being reached, and in developing new programmes. With its widespread network of institutions and large human resource base, the education sector may be better qualified than any other to gather, disseminate, and maintain this kind of information. The World Bank has supported the development of a sourcebook of this kind for developing countries, with special emphasis on sub-Saharan Africa (World Bank, 2003). There is room for a similar initiative in the Caribbean.

Supporting approaches through the media

The entertainment media, radio and television, are willingly accessed. What the media portray and discuss tends to have a very strong influence on the beliefs and attitudes of their audiences. Sometimes this influence is used in ways that are detrimental to the struggle with HIV/AIDS. Models frequently brought before audiences –

through advertisements, on television, and through the entertainment industry – glorify the physical aspects of sex, but say little about the arduous task of building enduring human relationships that support and are supported by sexual practice. 'While young people obtain a great deal of information about reproductive health from entertainment programmes in the mass media, many of these programmes have the effect of promoting attitudes and behaviour and portraying sex in ways that encourage risk-taking' (Kiragu, 2001: 18).

On the other hand, it needs to be recognised that if properly researched, designed and delivered, media and entertainment presentations can be powerful channels for the communication of correct information and the development of healthy attitudes. In this way they can have a significant role in influencing young people to adopt behaviour patterns that will protect them against HIV infection. A significantly important feature of this approach is its ability to reach large numbers on their own ground, including those who are not participating in any formal educational programme.

The education sector should be prepared to give its backing to television, radio, newspaper, booklet, entertainment and billboard presentations that are in harmony with its own efforts at HIV prevention education in schools and elsewhere. For the greater part, media professionals are the ones who should develop, produce and broadcast these materials, but preferably with input and advice from the education sector. The special nature of the Caribbean community, with small populations in many territories, a shared culture, and a strong culture of self-expression through music, suggests the desirability of some television and other productions with an HIV preventive education focus, designed for use throughout the region. This is an area that calls strongly for dynamic cooperation between the education sector and its many other partners. By adopting a proactive approach an education ministry would clearly manifest its concern that HIV prevention education reached all young people in its institutions and those outside the formal education system.

CHAPTER 10

HIV/AIDS and Tertiary Level Education

There are several reasons why every tertiary level education institution, especially those in a society affected by HIV/AIDS, must engage dynamically and proactively with the epidemic:

1. No institution is immune from the disease. In a society that experiences HIV/AIDS, no institution can regard itself as an AIDS-free enclave. Quite the contrary, a tertiary level institution may well be more severely affected than the surrounding society. This is because the great majority of the educational community in such an institution are young, in their late teens or early twenties, ages where the prevalence of HIV infection is particularly high. The risks are also heightened by the liberal atmosphere that tends to characterise institutions at this level and by campus cultures that may be open to activities, behaviours and life-styles that increase the possibility of HIV transmission.

2. Every institution has a responsibility for the well-being of those who are its members. At the tertiary level these comprise students, teaching and research staff, and all categories of employees. Three objectives should guide the work of the institution in discharging its responsibility for the well-being of all of these: to create an environment that reduces the likelihood of HIV transmission, to establish conditions that ensure that those with HIV and AIDS can safely reveal their

status and access appropriate support and counselling, and to provide care and support for those who are infected or affected by the disease.

3.   The disease has the potential to impair institutional functioning. The mechanisms through which HIV/AIDS undermines the operations of other institutions can also be at work at the higher educational level. The dynamics of the disease can manifest themselves in negative impacts on student numbers and learning potential, increased staff morbidity and mortality, reduced staff and student productivity, diversion of concerns and resources to coping or response measures, and increased financial costs.

4.   The long lead-time between initial HIV infection and the development of AIDS has major implications for tertiary level institutions. Some students may already be HIV infected by the time they commence programmes at this level and may become overtly ill during the time of their studies. For others, the real situation may not unfold until they have graduated and entered the world of work because the two to five years of most tertiary programmes may be too short a time for AIDS to manifest itself in those who were already HIV-infected when they entered the institution, or who became infected during the period of their studies or training. The institution may be successful in graduating qualified individuals, but HIV/AIDS can undermine its accomplishments by the premature deaths of young graduates. For those who remain permanently at the institution, including its academic and professional staff, the real impact, in the form of sicknesses and deaths, may not reveal itself for several years. Meanwhile the threat that the disease constitutes may seem unreal, leading to what amounts to practical denial that HIV/AIDS is an issue that the institution and each of its members need to take seriously.

5.   The mandate of service to society demands the engagement of every tertiary level education institution with HIV/AIDS. Tertiary level institutions exist so that they can meet society's need for knowledge, understanding and expertise, for the greater

part in well-defined specialised areas. In regions such as the Caribbean, where they serve societies in which HIV/AIDS has become a crucial public concern, these institutions are duty bound to respond to the needs of a society for HIV/AIDS-related scholarship and skills. In the circumstances of the epidemic, the leaders of these institutions and those who advise them or establish their policies must now include a specific HIV/AIDS response in their operational plans.

6.   Tertiary level institutions have a special responsibility for the development of human resources. These institutions are the principal agents for the preparation of a large segment of the professional and skilled personnel that society needs. In the context of HIV/AIDS, this imposes three responsibilities on them: (1) to ensure that all of the graduates from their programmes are competent to deal with HIV/AIDS, personally in their own lives and professionally in their area of expertise, where relevant; (2) to ensure that the institutions continue to produce graduates in the changing numbers needed by a society where the epidemic may be eroding the human resource base; and (3) to introduce new areas of professional training to respond to emerging needs in a society affected by the disease.

7.   Tertiary level institutions are crucial agents of change and providers of leadership directions for society. Whether one is talking about behaviour change, the eradication of stigma and discrimination, care and support for those infected or affected by the disease, or treatment for those who are ill, every successful response to HIV/AIDS requires new ways of going about things and the leadership that will guide and inspire individuals, communities and society to adopt those new ways. Every tertiary level education institution has a crucial role to play in this domain, serving as a role model, as a facilitator, and as the source of new knowledge, understanding and skills.

These issues are not merely theoretical. They reflect what is already occurring in Caribbean tertiary level institutions, although at the time of writing this does not appear to be widely appreciated. In various institutions there are students and staff who are living with HIV and AIDS. The attainment of personal and institutional goals is being compromised. In some institutions, individual and institutional responsibility to respond to the epidemic is gradually being acknowledged. In others, the reality of what is occurring is being ignored, played down, or denied.

The response of tertiary level education institutions to HIV/AIDS

These considerations highlight the problem and challenge that HIV/AIDS poses for every tertiary level education institution – the problem of responding to the needs of its own community given that, to a greater or less extent, it is an AIDS-affected institution; and the challenge of re-interpreting its core business in the AIDS-affected circumstances of society. They also point to the need for every institution to develop its own coordinated response to the epidemic, taking account of its clientele and area of expertise. For every institution, such a response will involve adaptations in its thinking, teaching and training functions, and in the way it manages itself. The response will also depend very heavily on the commitment of the institution's leaders and senior executives.

Tertiary level curriculum change in response to HIV/AIDS.

It is generally agreed that the curriculum in every tertiary level institution must incorporate HIV/AIDS and related issues. There is less agreement, however, on the rationale for such curriculum adaptation. The curriculum incorporation of HIV/AIDS is seen as bringing at least two types of benefits to students – the personal and the professional.

- The personal benefits are the knowledge, skills, attitudes and values that can come from tertiary level HIV/AIDS education. Although much may have been accomplished in secondary school, students at the higher level need wider and more profound understanding appropriate to their level of education.

The expectation is that expanding their practical and theoretical understanding of HIV/AIDS will equip them for the reduction of HIV transmission, the provision of care and support, and the mitigation of adverse impacts.

- The professional benefits are that students will be better equipped to work in an AIDS-affected society. The aim would be to ensure that they develop a very clear professional understanding of the epidemic, how it impacts on their area of study or training, how it affects the world of work in general and in their chosen area of expertise, and hence what it is likely to mean in terms of their future careers.

Not many universities and other tertiary level institutions have clarified for themselves which of these approaches they should adopt, whether HIV/AIDS programmes at the tertiary level should be 'prevention driven' or 'profession driven'. Some institutions have introduced compulsory courses that deal with HIV/AIDS in a conventional higher education framework of lectures, research, assignments, and tests, but with the primary purpose of equipping students to make better choices in their social and sexual relationships (ACU, 2002: 27). Others have adopted a different model, preferring to leave it to the various departments to ensure the integration of HIV/AIDS into the professional training programmes.

There are good reasons for and against both approaches. An HIV/AIDS course which all students must complete as part of their academic requirements would be an unequivocal statement of institutional concern. It would bring the HIV/AIDS issue out into the open, ensure that the appropriate messages reach all students, and serve as a channel for dispelling ignorance and misunderstanding. On the other hand, the establishment of such a required general course could obstruct the mainstreaming of HIV/AIDS into specific professional programmes since it could create the misconception that sufficient attention had already been paid to the topic. Further concerns about an institution-wide compulsory course relate to the danger of superficiality, given that such a course would have to cover so much in what would necessarily be a relatively short period of time; possible student resistance and 'AIDS fatigue'; and the questionable value of a generalised course coming late in a student's life (individual need for such a course would have been experienced several years earlier, close to the onset of puberty or in early adolescence).

A compromise position would be to seek to produce graduates who are competent to manage and control HIV/AIDS within their respective areas of professional training, but to ensure that the programmes that bring this about provide students with knowledge, understanding and skills that they could use to their personal benefit in protecting themselves against HIV risks and in making informed and life-protecting choices. The primary aim would be professional AIDS-competence and the secondary aim personal HIV protection. AIDS-competence refers to a theoretical and practical understanding of the epidemic, appropriate to the programme of study being undertaken, and its implications for the future careers of participating students. In promoting AIDS-competence, the purpose would be to develop in students a mature understanding of the epidemic, the aspects of it that they are likely to encounter in their subsequent professional lives, and to equip them with some tools and skills for addressing it within their areas of professional expertise.

This professional understanding will have another component, which is that as many graduating students as possible will have been fully trained in the management, political, social, economic and legal aspects of AIDS in the workplace. They will be able to generate workplace programmes that include peer education and counselling, as well as understanding of the relevant legislation and the effects of large numbers of sick and dying colleagues (Crewe, 2000: 120).

Looking at this from the perspective of students, it is probably the case that most students expect that their education and training will help them to succeed in the working world. In a world with HIV/AIDS, making them AIDS-competent should contribute positively to this.

Integrating HIV/AIDS in this way into the professional aspects of the curriculum requires that the teaching staff develop a good general understanding of the epidemic and its effects, in addition to specific understanding of the interaction between HIV/AIDS and the area of professional expertise. Hence, a critical priority in the response of a tertiary level institution to HIV/AIDS is to ensure the development of the necessary staff competence. If they are to develop AIDS-competent students, staff themselves must be AIDS-competent. Through in-house and inter-institutional training sessions, every member of staff must understand the epidemic in ways that exceed even an educated public. Through special training and self-development opportunities, staff within respective disciplines need to develop a clear understanding and knowledge of specific aspects of HIV/AIDS in the workplace where their graduates will be employed, and to be aware of the relevant precautions, support and care provisions.

The Health Economics and HIV/AIDS Research Division (HEARD) at the University of Natal, South Africa, has developed a number of AIDS toolkits and briefs designed to help in the development of sector-specific responses to the epidemic and to alert sector managers to various HIV/AIDS-related issues within different sectors. While the perspective is that of southern Africa, these materials can assist curriculum planners in recognising HIV/AIDS implications in a variety of professional and training areas. The AIDS briefs for professionals and for sectoral planners and managers might serve as initial resource material for such training.[1]

Institutional management

The institutionalisation of HIV/AIDS within the teaching programmes of tertiary level institutions needs to be accompanied and supported by its institutionalisation at the level of management. Every aspect of the disease must be factored into the management arrangements. Because of the long lead-time between infection and any visible sign of illness, the disease can be working away silently in an institution, with the possibility of high levels of HIV infection among students and eventual progression to AIDS among staff.

Planning and management arrangements have to take this into account.

At the management level there is need to attend to the following:

- The mobilisation of HIV awareness and institution-wide commitment to dealing with the problem among all sectors of the community – students, teaching and professional staff and support staff.

- A review of policies governing the admission, progression, and performance of students, and the employment, promotion, and performance of staff, to ensure that they take full account of HIV/AIDS and do not discriminate in any way against any individual who has been infected or affected by the disease.

- Meeting the needs of management and finance departments for good information about the manifestations and progress of the disease among students and staff.

- Arrangements for meeting the direct and indirect costs arising from the disease.

- A review of policies and procedures governing medical insurance, sick leave, loans, benefits, and pensions, to ensure that they are appropriate in the circumstances of HIV/AIDS.

- Where prevalence levels are high, procedures for the speedy recruitment and training of replacement staff.

At the level of social and working relations in the institution there is need to consider:

- Establishing partnerships with staff and students that will rally the involvement of the institution's entire community in fostering HIV prevention, care and support for the infected or affected, and initiatives to manage negative impacts.

- The engagement of all campus cultures and groups – students, staff, language, religious, entertainment and other associations, and societies – in the common struggle against the disease. Among these, particular importance is attached to student governing bodies and religious associations.

- How to respond to values and practices in campus life that may facilitate HIV transmission.

- Provision of health, counselling, and testing services. Three special areas of concern are ensuring adequate services and supplies for treating STIs, ensuring access to adequately resourced facilities for the treatment of opportunistic infections (pneumonia, TB, thrush, etc.), and providing for voluntary counselling and testing (VCT).

- Making special provision for HIV prevention, treatment, and care (including issues relating to the provision of antiretrovirals).

- Protecting the right to privacy and ensuring that strict confidentiality is maintained in relation to all information about the medical condition or sexual history of a member of the institutional community.

- Occupational safety procedures for students, academic staff and support staff.

- Workplace education for staff, in accordance with the ILO recommendation that workplace information and education programmes be adopted as essential in combating the spread of the epidemic and contributing to the capacity of workers to protect themselves against HIV infection (ILO, 2001: 9).

- Challenging denial and stigma, and reducing HIV-related anxiety.

Institutional leadership

The response of a tertiary level institution to HIV/AIDS depends very heavily on the commitment of its leaders and senior executives. If there is a totally dedicated, committed leadership, the response is likely to succeed in its aims. In the absence of such leadership it is likely to falter. In some institutions, individuals are already taking steps in their responses to the demands of the epidemic. In most situations, however, the responses are from rank and file individuals within the institutions. As such, they do not constitute a bona fide institutional response. Reports from all parts of the world, including the Caribbean, are unanimous in affirming that committed leadership at a high level is the most critical factor for driving a strong institutional response to HIV/AIDS. Given the right leadership it is possible to inspire key stakeholders, mobilise resources, establish policies, and set up management structures. Above all, it is possible to demonstrate that until the disease has been overcome, responding creatively and proactively to HIV/AIDS will feature prominently among institutional concerns.

This personal commitment on the part of the institution's top leadership should translate into a total management commitment that manifests itself in:

- an authoritative strategic planning and policy development approach;
- the commitment of resources;
- the establishment of the necessary implementation structures within an appropriate institutional framework;
- a sustained challenge to all forms of on-campus denial, stigma and discrimination, accompanied by steps to facilitate HIV openness;
- efforts to ensure that every official of lesser rank implements institutional policies, strategies and interventions aimed at the control of the disease and the mitigation of its personal and institutional impacts; and
- well-developed accountability arrangements that facilitate the identification of bottlenecks or sluggishness in the implementation of institutional plans for responding to the epidemic.

The special role of certain key institutions

Every tertiary level education institution plays an important role in the struggle with HIV/AIDS – internally by striving to protect its students and staff and thereby its own functioning, and externally by adjusting its education programmes in response to the needs of an AIDS-affected society. The internal responsibility towards students, staff and self-preservation as a functioning institution is shared by every institution. However, the nature of certain institutions, and the scope of their operations, accentuate their responsibility to look to the needs of society. In the Caribbean these strategically placed institutions would include universities, teachers' colleges and education institutes, and theology colleges for the preparation of church pastors.

Universities

Universities and reflection on HIV/AIDS

The first responsibility of a university in relation to HIV/AIDS is to be in the forefront in developing deeper understandings of it, as a disease, an epidemic, a psycho-social phenomenon and an intellectual challenge. Although prominent on the world scene for more than two decades, HIV/AIDS is far from being fully understood. Increased knowledge of HIV as a virus and of AIDS as a biomedical condition has led to the development of antiretroviral therapies and may in time lead to the development of therapeutic and prevention vaccines. However, there has been no corresponding growth in understanding HIV/AIDS as a social phenomenon. The disease continues to flourish behind a wall of silence, while fear of stigma and discrimination prevents its being brought out into the open. The discourse of AIDS is characterised by a language of conflict and struggle that works in synergy with a language of exclusion, leading to a dehumanisation of affected or infected individuals and a marginalisation of HIV/AIDS concerns. For over two decades, information, communication and education campaigns have attempted to influence AIDS-relevant behaviour, but failed because they were based on inappropriate communication models and did not take adequate account of cultural and spiritual values (UNAIDS, 1999b).

Universities are well positioned to deal with these and similar issues as a result of their intellectual resources and traditions. In many respects they are the thinking-caps of society which provides them with resources and the freedom to do the hard work of reflection on its behalf. In relation to HIV/AIDS, they are challenged to dedicate their best efforts to unravelling the many layers of understanding that enwrap the disease so that humanity can come to terms with its intellectual, philosophical, theological, linguistic, and other dimensions. Thereby efforts to prevent and manage it can become more tractable and successful. A publication from the University of the West Indies has performed signal service in this regard (Howe and Cobley, 2000). The Caribbean and the academic world await further manifestations of the widespread engagement of Caribbean universities with the overall intellectual challenge posed by HIV/ AIDS.

HIV/AIDS and the preparation of university graduates

In addition, universities in the Caribbean have a major responsibility to respond to HIV/AIDS in the fields of human resource development, research and strategic engagement with society. This has been well expressed by the University of the West Indies in its HIV/AIDS Response Programme (UWI HARP) (*Box 21*).

Box 21. The University of the West Indies HIV/ AIDS response programme (UWI HARP)

The **mission** of UWI HARP is to help build and use the capacities of the University in order to add to an interdisciplinary understanding of HIV/AIDS, to contribute substantially to HIV/ AIDS prevention and care, and to help mitigate the impact of the HIV/AIDS epidemic.

The **aims** of the programme are to:

1. Accelerate action by UWI in response to the growing HIV/ AIDS epidemic through research, education, and training, and strategic engagement with the wider society.

2. Develop and monitor HIV/AIDS policies.

Box 21 (cont'd).

3. Generate/attract/manage resources to sustain the response to HIV/AIDS.

4. Serve as a clearinghouse for HIV/AIDS information, working in partnership with and complementing national, regional and international agencies.

Source: UWI HARP Strategic Planning Workshop Report, August 2002.

Universities, in the Caribbean as elsewhere, are duty bound to respond to the challenge posed by this situation and to ensure the development of skilled personnel in the areas needed and in the numbers required. This may necessitate new programmes, new fields of training and inquiry, cross-disciplinary teaching, innovative methods for programme delivery, collaborative teaching between institutions, the involvement of non-university partners in the design and delivery of programmes, and adjustment in student numbers.

In keeping with these perspectives, the University of the West Indies (UWI) has adopted an imaginative and proactive framework for substantial curriculum development. UWI aims at advancing its response to HIV/AIDS through a set of curriculum development priorities identified in a wide-ranging consultation process (*Box 22*). Some of these are inward looking and relate to needs within UWI itself; others are outward looking and are aimed at preparing appropriately skilled professionals to contribute to the prevention of HIV infection and the mitigation of the effects of the epidemic on the individual and on society. An important aspect of the process was the care taken to ensure that the proposed priorities were consistent with areas identified in the Caribbean Regional Plan of Action for HIV/AIDS. The priorities cover health and life sciences, social sciences and law, and communications.

Box 22. UWI priority curriculum and programming responses to HIV/AIDS

Cross cutting priorities

1. For all UWI academic staff of all faculties and institutes on all campuses and NCC centres: Increase sensitisation to the HIV/AIDS epidemic and to the response required of the university.

2. Ensure that every person in the UWI community has the knowledge and behaviour to protect herself/himself from contracting HIV.

3. Ensure that institutional and individual behaviour toward people living with HIV/AIDS (PLA) is dignified and humanitarian.

Health/life sciences priorities

4. Ensure that new-generation health care practitioners graduate, fully able to contribute to HIV/AIDS prevention and care. (Reference to health care practitioners includes medical doctors, dentists, all categories of nurses, medical social workers and persons in the allied health professions).

5. Ensure that older-generation health care practitioners become HIV/AIDS-capable.

6. Prepare a cadre of epidemic prevention and mitigation managers to augment the leadership of regional and national programmes of HIV/AIDS prevention and control.

7. Ensure that among graduating life scientists there is a cohort with in-depth knowledge of HIV/AIDS, who are willing to contribute to research, training of other professionals and public education.

8. Prepare a cadre of nurse educators and administrators to facilitate national delivery of training for nursing assistants to care peripatetically for terminally ill home-based patients.

Box 22 (cont'd).

Social sciences/law priorities

9. Ensure that new-generation law graduates are sensitive to reforms in Caribbean legislation that will contribute to the containment of the HIV/AIDS epidemic.

10. Provide new undergraduate/graduate courses in psychology and behaviour change and new courses focussed on international/ Caribbean consequences of the HIV/AIDS epidemic for economies, societies, security and governance.

11. Develop a new certificated course for HIV/AIDS Infection Prevention and Support Counsellors, to include trainees who are HIV positive.

Communication priorities

12. Develop degree programmes in health communication. This should include the stimulation and encouragement of research to develop in-depth knowledge and new insights to replace or enrich traditional approaches to communication for behaviour change.

13. Develop and publish instructional resources for effective promotion of HIV/AIDS prevention behaviour among upper primary level students.

14. Develop a curriculum on theology, epidemics and the role of faith-based organisations.

Source: Bain and Morrissey, 2002: 5.

The development of the UWI proposals brings out how the response must match the characteristics of the virus and how, as is repeated so often, with HIV/AIDS it can no longer be business as usual. HIV/AIDS is challenging universities to be as all-encompassing, flexible and innovative in their response as the virus is in its attack.

In addition, it is challenging them to have a sense of urgency in their response and to commit themselves wholeheartedly to ensuring that the region has the skilled human resources needed to assure success in the combat with the epidemic.

In more general terms, universities in the Caribbean that seek to enhance their response to HIV/AIDS-generated human resource needs in the region should take account of the following four dimensions:

1.   By integrating HIV/AIDS issues across existing programmes or introducing special HIV/AIDS courses, they should ensure that every programme provides for rigorous scientific reflection on the epidemic. This is with a view to ensuring that all of their students become AIDS-competent at a depth that befits university graduates.

2.   Recognising that in a world with AIDS, graduates need greater flexibility so that they can more readily assume roles and responsibilities for which they may not have been explicitly prepared, every programme should seek to adjust its teaching methodologies to foster more independent and self-motivated learning. This will help to equip students with the intellectual tools that will enable them to be more adaptable and innovative in responding to the needs of a fast-changing and unpredictable world with AIDS.

3.   Faculties and departments should consider the need to introduce new areas of emphasis or explore areas where the epidemic demands a shift in emphasis. Express efforts should be made to introduce HIV/AIDS-related issues into various social science, legal, and humanities programmes. A need has already been identified for developments of this kind in such widely diverging areas as health economics, responding to the challenge of orphans, dealing with ethical issues, theoretical and practical understanding of community mobilisation,[2] policy analysis, communication strategies for behaviour change, decentralisation, bereavement counselling, and the role of cultural determinants in the formation of values, attitudes and behaviours.

4.   Institutions should consider the need to increase student numbers in areas where HIV/AIDS is eroding society's skills

base and also in areas where it is foreseen that because of the epidemic there will be a need in future years for an increasing number of qualified individuals (as has already been recognised in many of the social and para-medical areas).

Universities and HIV/AIDS research

In the area of research, the challenge for universities is clear: undertake more HIV/AIDS-related research. New knowledge is critical to efforts at understanding, combating and managing the epidemic. Responding to this imperative touches on a university's core business to generate and disseminate new knowledge. Their dense concentration of intellectual expertise makes universities particularly well equipped to do so. Society has invested heavily in them so that they can develop, elaborate and evaluate knowledge through study; expand and generate it through research; and disseminate and spread it through publications and conferences. Hence universities in the region must be at the cutting edge in the search for improved bio-medical, epidemiological, scientific, social and economic understandings of HIV/AIDS. They are duty bound to make their own unique contribution to the various areas of prevention, care and support, treatment and impact management. Thereby they will contribute significantly to improvements in the quality of life for an appreciable number of human beings.

In June 2001, the UN General Assembly Special Session on HIV/AIDS underlined the importance of research when it stated that 'with no cure for HIV/AIDS yet found, further research and development are crucial' (UNGASS, 2001: 22). The Assembly also called for increased investment in HIV/AIDS-related research and development, including biomedical operations, and social, cultural and behavioural research (Article 70). More specifically, in words that could have been written with the Caribbean in mind, the United Nations called for numerous research-related developments in 'those countries experiencing or at risk of a rapid expansion of the epidemic' (Article 71). The programmes envisaged relate to the development of national and international research infrastructure, laboratory capacity, improved surveillance systems, data collection, processing and dissemination, and training of basic and clinical researchers, social scientists, health-care providers and technicians.

A few simple principles can serve to guide the HIV/AIDS research portfolio of a university:

- Because HIV/AIDS is a multi-dimensional development issue and not just a health issue, much HIV/AIDS research will be characterised by teamwork involving researchers from the biomedical, pure science and social science fields. Good HIV/AIDS research work will regularly transcend disciplinary boundaries and, at the very least, will take account of findings from a broad spectrum of investigations.

- HIV/AIDS is an area of investigation that lends itself particularly well to collaborative efforts between universities themselves (within the region and internationally), and between universities and various bodies in society. The Caribbean is richly resourced with a variety of national and regional bodies with an interest in research on HIV/AIDS. The research undertakings of these institutions can be more purposefully directed through cooperation and collaboration. UNICA, the Association of Caribbean Universities and Research Institutes, has the mandate of facilitating academic contacts and collaborative work and supports the regionalisation of higher education in the Caribbean. As such, it is uniquely well placed to promote collaborative research between its member universities. The added value of such cooperation would be increased understanding of HIV/AIDS in multinational, multilinguistic, and multicultural settings. Other important partners for university cooperation, at both regional and national levels, include CAREC, the Caribbean Regional Epidemiological Centre; CRN+, the Caribbean Network of People Living with HIV/AIDS; CHRC, the Caribbean Regional Health Council; various members of the United Nations family; the multilateral and bilateral agencies; and regional and international NGOs.

- Because the impacts of HIV/AIDS on individual human well-being and on development broadly understood are so devastating and all-encompassing, HIV/AIDS research should keep the end users constantly in view. Until the world can demonstrate greater success in the battle with AIDS, the concern of AIDS-related research should focus less on the production of knowledge for its own sake, and more on how the new knowledge will contribute to the development of goods and services that will promote HIV prevention, sustain support and care, and mitigate adverse impacts.

- Mechanisms for the dissemination and sharing of research findings should be integral to every HIV/AIDS-related research proposal. In the absence of these mechanisms little can be done to utilise or further develop the newly generated knowledge. Universities and research institutions should ensure extensive use of traditional and emerging IT (information technology) channels for the rapid communication of their research findings.

The medical, health and life sciences are areas that stand in clear need of university-based HIV/AIDS research. But there is scope for HIV/AIDS-related research of the highest quality in such other areas as health economics; comprehensive assessments of impact in various sectors; the social sciences, especially psychology, counselling and care, and issues relating to the orphans challenge; ways of expanding the involvement of grassroots organisations and helping communities to cope; understanding and promoting traditional, alternative, and non-western approaches to health care, HIV prevention and AIDS treatment; the many legal implications of the disease and the status of legislative measures; ethical and human rights issues; philosophical and theological perspectives; communications approaches; computer modelling of the course of the epidemic and its economic and other impacts. The increase in international resources for responding to the epidemic points in another direction for university-level research – studies that monitor and evaluate the extent to which resources reach and benefit those most directly affected by the epidemic.

Universities and engagement with society

The final area of university responsibility is that of strategic engagement with society. Every university needs to develop a network of working relations with the various organs of society in the public and private sectors. These look to the universities to help them meet their human resource needs and to provide them with better practices, more profound understandings and new knowledge. But the traffic is not all one-way. Universities must also go to society in a learning capacity, especially in the area of HIV/AIDS. This is a new area of human experience where agencies, communities and private individuals may well be better informed, especially on details, than the university. This points to the learning role of the university in its engagement with society. It cannot afford to be arrogant and to act as if it were the controller and sole dispenser of knowledge. Instead it must work respectfully with agencies, communities and individuals, seeking jointly with them to identify the problems that need to be addressed and working jointly with them in finding solutions for these problems.

This has practical consequences for university teaching, research and community outreach programmes:

- It is highly desirable that AIDS-related engagement with and service to society be incorporated into student programme requirements. The needs of an AIDS-affected society are too grave to be left either to chance or to individual interest. University students who are required by their programmes to serve society in the AIDS domain proclaim loud and clear that the university is serious in its intention to engage with and overcome the epidemic. The knowledge and skills that students would develop when providing this service should later increase their marketability, since in an AIDS-affected society employers attach special value to those with some experience in coping with and managing the disease and its impacts.

- It is equally desirable that in its communication with society, the university goes out of its way to ensure the involvement of persons living with HIV/AIDS (PLAs), whether these be members of the university community or of the wider society. PLAs can contribute insights and articulate needs at depths that those who are not infected cannot plumb.

- Procedures for staff advancement should also pay special attention to evidence on the AIDS-related accomplishments of a member of staff in working with communities, government departments, non-governmental agencies, and other bodies. Once again, attaching special value to these is eloquent testimony that a university wishes to match its expressions of concern by action that will spur extensive involvement of its staff in working with others for the prevention, control and management of HIV/AIDS.

The crucial point therefore, is that the university should care about HIV/AIDS within its own ranks and in the society it serves, and show that it cares. In today's world, universities are judged by the variety and vitality of their interactions with the societies of which they are part (ACU, 2001). In a region such as the Caribbean, where the HIV prevalence rates are alarmingly high, they will be especially judged by the dynamism of their interactions with society in the field of HIV/AIDS.

Teachers' colleges and education institutes

There are three areas where teachers' colleges and education institutes (including those located within universities) are called upon to play a critical role in the struggle with HIV/AIDS: the preparation of teachers in the composite area of HIV/AIDS, sexual and reproductive health, and life skills; the development and production of instructional materials for this area; and quality assurance for field programmes (including support for the ongoing professional development of serving teachers). If the colleges and institutes do not assume responsibility in these areas, teacher preparation, the development of instructional materials, and quality assurance will go by default, meaningful HIV/AIDS-related education in schools will remain a myth, and succeeding generations of young people will not receive the help they need (and that could be provided) to prepare them for a world with HIV/AIDS.

The initial professional training programme needs to ensure that every newly qualified teacher is AIDS-competent in two respects:

- Each newly qualified teacher has the knowledge and understanding needed by a teacher who is to teach at a given level; and

- each newly qualified teacher is psychologically comfortable with teaching AIDS and sexuality issues to children and adolescents, both boys and girls.

This implies that the training programme must deal with three areas:

1. Imparting the knowledge, understanding and skills that have to be acquired for successful teaching about HIV/AIDS, sexual and reproductive health, and life-skills.

2. Developing teaching methodologies and instructional skills for this area of concern.

3. Addressing the taboos, stigma, anxieties, and psychological blockages that stand in the way of effective teaching in these areas.

In addition, there should be provision for some trainees to become more specialised in these areas. Even in the most optimistic scenarios, HIV/AIDS will remain as a global problem for several decades into the future, and hence a major concern for schools as they admit successive generations of pupils. It is imperative, therefore, that relevant education programmes be professionalised, with the concentrated preparation of a number of teachers specialised in HIV/AIDS-related areas who will be able to provide support for teachers with a more general level of preparation.

Colleges and institutes must also concern themselves with the development of the necessary instructional resources. The inadequacy of such resources is undermining HFLE efforts. If the needs are not met, HIV/AIDS, sexuality education, and life-skills will continue to be relegated to the sidelines. Together with serving teachers, the colleges and institutes know the schools and their needs better than others do. They are also intimately acquainted with what is good and not so good in the area of textbooks, workbooks and other instructional resources. What they need is to apply all this knowledge and deep understanding to developing, in cooperation with teachers, materials relating to HIV/AIDS, sexual and reproductive health, and life-skills. The adolescent-friendly summary of research studies on adolescents in Jamaica (UNICEF/UNFPA, 2002) shows what can be done. Given the size of the potential market and the likelihood of long-term needs, local publishers would almost certainly support the development of similar materials. The colleges and institutes should feel challenged to take the lead in an area that could be crucial to the success of Caribbean countries in their struggle with HIV/AIDS.

A final challenge to the colleges and institutes is to contribute to ensuring the maintenance and, if necessary, the improvement of the quality of teaching about HIV/AIDS and related subjects that is already being provided in schools. A major contribution would be to participate in bringing all serving teachers up to a minimum standard in this area. This would almost certainly involve a wide range of inservice programmes and on-the-job training for serving teachers. Clearly there would be a need for education ministries to be heavily involved in this (and to mobilise the necessary resources). But the problem is so large that ministries may defer action unless stimulated by proposals from colleges and institutes. A further contribution would be to provide more intensive and somewhat specialised training for ministry quality assurance personnel, so that they in turn can be more effective in monitoring what the schools are doing in the area of HIV/AIDS education and be more supportive in their advice to teachers. The aim should be to ensure that the composite area of HIV/AIDS, sexual and reproductive health, and life-skills, is fully professionalised, has a school status comparable to that of other disciplines, and is adequately catered for in the timetable, in the allocation of resources for instructional and library materials, and in the actual teaching.

Theology colleges for the preparation of pastors

Churches and faith-based organisations are organs of considerable significance in the Caribbean. The importance of the church to people is highlighted by the case of Jamaica where it is alleged that there are more church buildings per person than in any other part of the world. The pastors who minister to their people in the wide network of Caribbean churches and faith-based communities constitute a vitally important force in the struggle with HIV/AIDS. They have extensive reserves of strength, followers and commitment that give them significant advantages in delivering HIV/AIDS messages and interventions. In addition to being respected leaders within their respective communities, they have privileged access to various groups, including those in school, the sick in their homes or in hospital, the armed forces, and those in prison. 'In addition, their jurisdiction often includes a number of areas closely connected to HIV/AIDS, such as morality, beliefs about the spiritual bases of disease, and rules of family life and sexual activity' (Liebowitz, 2002: 2).

Because HIV/AIDS will certainly be an important pastoral concern for them in their later ministry, and because of their potential to spearhead much of the community mobilisation needed for confronting the epidemic, HIV/AIDS should be integral to the training programme of every future pastor. AIDS-competence is as important for them as it is for university graduates and for future teachers. The learning needs of pastors have never been extensively considered, possibly because the training remained so exclusively within the realms of the faith-based communities themselves. But the need exists to support those communities in ensuring that their future spiritual leaders, who will be men and women of great influence among them, have an adequate understanding of HIV/AIDS, learn how to deal with it pastorally and compassionately, and recognise their potential to provide their communities with resources and hope in the struggle against HIV/AIDS.

Achieving this would be expedited if programmes of pastoral study and formation in theological colleges and similar institutions ensured:

- the integration of HIV/AIDS concerns and pastoral experiences into the programmes of formation for future pastors;
- the appropriate integration of HIV/AIDS into their programmes of study;
- special attention during their period of formation to issues of major concern, such as orphans, HIV-based stigma and discrimination, home-based care, violence and sexual abuse, constructive responses to youth needs, and the strengthening of the family;
- the development of new perspectives in the theology of hope, grief and suffering, morality, gender, and poverty.

It would help also if the theological colleges could do for serving pastors what it is proposed the teacher colleges should do for serving teachers – that is, reach out to them to make them AIDS-aware and AIDS-competent, through seminars, meetings, the production and dissemination of suitable literature, and the establishment of networks for information sharing on practices, interventions, issues, and needs.

Notes

1.   AIDS toolkits are available for finance, health, housing and public works, labour, and welfare. AIDS briefs for professionals are available for advertisers, architects, human resource managers, insurance personnel, media personnel, politicians, religious leaders, social workers, the legal profession, town and regional planners. AIDS briefs for sectoral planners and managers are available for sectors such as the civil service, commercial agricultural, construction, education, fisheries industry, health, the informal sector, life assurance industry, manufacturing, media, military, mining, oil industry, prisons, social sector, sports, tourism, transport, and trade unions. Documents can be downloaded from the HEARD web site www.und.ac.za/und/heard.

2.   "Community mobilisation is the core strategy on which success against HIV has been built" (UNAIDS, 2002a: 16).

STRATEGIC APPROACHES: A SUMMARY

CHAPTER 11

Ten Lines of Action

'Education can be a powerful force – perhaps the most powerful force of all – in combating the spread of HIV/AIDS' (UNESCO, 2000: 22-23). Education authorities across the Caribbean, especially the top level political and management authorities, need firm convictions on this score. Those outside the education sector also need to see the education sector operating to its full potential and proving that it really is a powerful force in the struggle against HIV/AIDS. By adopting certain strategic lines of action (*Box 23*), the education sector in the region will ensure that it can meet this challenge.

Box 23. Ten strategic lines of action for the education sector in the Caribbean

1. Develop a regional response through the education sector.
2. Keep HIV/AIDS high in the educational dialogue across the region and in the various countries.
3. Underpin regional planning for HIV/AIDS in education with corresponding planning, policy and capacity development at the national level.
4. Forge multisectoral and multilevel partnerships at regional and national levels.

Box 23 (cont'd).

5. Base the sector's approach on the three basic strategies of prevention, care and support, and impact mitigation within the sector.

6. Make full use of the region's cultural diversity for a better understanding of the problem and ways of addressing it.

7. Ensure that every policy and procedure is firmly rooted in human rights and that every feature of the education sector manifests a strong human rights approach.

8. Ensure that gender dimensions are fully integrated in all policies, procedures and programmes of instruction.

9. Pay specific attention to the attainment of the UNGASS targets for prevention, information and orphan assistance.

10. Use the opportunity presented by the HIV/AIDS crisis to strengthen the education sector's ability to develop the 'ideal Caribbean person'.

Develop a regional education response

The Caribbean is a large multilingual region of great cultural richness and social and economic diversity. Within the framework of this diversity, the region experiences a strong sense of unity based on historical developments, the ancestral origins of its people, features of trade and commerce, and formal and informal alliances of Caribbean people within and outside the region. The 'unified diversity' that is the Caribbean has given rise to CARICOM, the Caribbean Community which brings together the independent states and dependencies in the Caribbean (with the exception of Cuba) for the promotion of trade and cooperation in many areas. The CARICOM Heads of Government gave eloquent expression to this unity of the Caribbean community when, in 1997, they adopted the profile of the 'ideal Caribbean person' (*Box 26*).

Education is seen as playing a crucial role in the development of this holistic Caribbean person. But the variety of HIV epidemics throughout the region jeopardises its ability to do so. These can only be addressed by a region-wide educational response, in addition to the national level action that is proposed below. Some specific considerations underline the importance of a regional education response to HIV/AIDS:

- Educational leaders throughout the region need to be guided by a common vision of the dynamic interaction between education and HIV/AIDS, each with the potential to undermine the other.

- Strategies and action programmes for an educational response to HIV/AIDS across the region necessarily have many features in common.

- For many undertakings, resource mobilisation can be more successful if based on understanding and planning that transcend national considerations.

- The dynamic interaction between the countries of the region, which are so energetically expressed in the freedom with which Caribbean people (including their children) move from one country to another, demand a common educational response to the epidemic.

- Many of the interventions required in the education sector place heavy demands on human capacity. By acting in unison, the many small states in the region would be better placed to provide for human capacity needs than when acting alone.

- A regional education response can be implemented through existing regional institutions, such as UWI or the Pan-Caribbean Partnership Against AIDS (PANCAP), or can be coordinated by bodies that serve regional needs, such as UNESCO's office for the Caribbean.

The CARICOM Health and Family Life Education (HFLE) initiative is a practical expression of regional cooperation in education. This initiative merits further development and extension to all

Caribbean countries, with curriculum and materials development being reviewed in the light of developing understandings on effective HIV/AIDS communication strategies (*Chapters 4 and 6*) and greater emphasis on ensuring that all new and serving teachers are suitably equipped to deliver HIV prevention education and to contribute within their schools and communities to mitigating the effects of the epidemic.

Other areas that call for a larger measure of regional cooperation include:

- The development of capacity across the entire education sector to maximise the impact of education on HIV/AIDS and to minimise the impact of HIV/AIDS on education.
- The development of AIDS-competent teachers and support for them in their work.
- The development of policies and procedures for dealing with HIV positive educators and/or learners, including regulations governing medical assistance and various benefits.
- Possible legislative measures and the harmonisation of educational HIV/AIDS provisions with international and national law.
- Developing ethical guidelines for impact assessments and other forms of HIV/AIDS-related educational research.
- Conducting impact assessments and other forms of research.
- The development of tools for regional use in assessing the impacts of HIV/AIDS on the sector (similar to, but going beyond, the Rapid Appraisal Framework presented in *Appendix 2*).
- The development of tools for regional use in such areas as projecting AIDS impacts on educator and learner numbers, orphan numbers, and additional AIDS costs to systems.
- The establishment of networks and other means for creating and sharing data, best practices, and various forms of information.

- The establishment of a regional task team of experts in HIV/ AIDS and education whose competence and knowledge would be available to education sectors throughout the region.

- Strengthening the potential of regional tertiary level institutions to respond to HIV/AIDS-needs in the fields of curriculum, materials, educational management and planning, and psycho-social counselling.

The enumeration of these areas suggests the desirability of establishing a pan-Caribbean organisation or network on HIV/AIDS and education that would concern itself with policy, planning, training, research and information needs. However, the success of such a venture would be heavily dependent on initial political support at the highest level, sustained commitment of the necessary resources, and the cooperation of relevant regional and internal organisations. Strong political support has been expressed in the assurance of the Caribbean Ministers of Education in the Havana Commitment (*Appendix 1*) that they would work 'for a regional approach in the framework of the Pan-Caribbean Partnership Against AIDS' and their request to UNESCO to assist PANCAP in establishing a regional forum on HIV/AIDS and education. Resource commitment and the involvement of regional and international organisations remain outstanding.

Ensure sustained advocacy for HIV/AIDS and education issues

The best projections are that HIV/AIDS is set to remain as a major global problem for another half century. Its historical development, mobility patterns within the Caribbean, and the importance to the region of the tourist industry, mean that it will also remain a major regional problem, with considerable likelihood that its salience for countries and for the region will increase. If education is to play a key role in what seems likely to be a protracted and more intensified struggle with the epidemic, then advocacy, sensitisation and awareness-building must be sustained as central concerns. There can be no room for 'AIDS fatigue', no allowing HIV/AIDS issues to be crowded off the agenda, no ignoring of the incessant calls of the epidemic for a meaningful response.

The first priority area named in the Caribbean Regional Strategic Plan of Action for HIV/AIDS is advocacy (together with policy development and legislation). It is similar with national plans from other parts of the world. It should likewise be similar for education throughout the region. Effective strategies for the use of education in the combat with HIV/AIDS require committed and informed leadership and the collective dedication of a wide range of partners. Mobilising this leadership and dedication requires advocacy. Maintaining it requires sustained advocacy. Persons from within the education sector must be seen and heard alongside their colleagues from health and other areas as credible advocates for a relevant and sustained response to HIV/AIDS.

There is need for sustained efforts to ensure that political authorities, especially those concerned with education, are kept aware of HIV/AIDS and education issues, of what the epidemic is doing to the sector, and what the sector's response is. The need to sustain such advocacy becomes all the more important because the epidemic seems set to endure for such a long time. Political changes will almost inevitably occur within that time and with them the possibility of changes in priorities. Sustained advocacy will ensure that, whatever the changes, HIV/AIDS remains a high priority for the education sector until the disease and its impacts have been vanquished.

Core tasks for sustained advocacy throughout the region and across the sector include:

- Securing the wholehearted support of political authorities, civic and religious leaders, and prominent citizens for the mainstreaming of HIV/AIDS into various facets of educational development and provision.

- Increasing the understanding that education's role extends beyond HIV prevention to include care and support for the infected and affected.

- Mobilising all educational institutions to play their role in HIV education along a continuum running from prevention to care.

- Winning the understanding and support of the regional and national media and entertainment industries for efforts directed to HIV education.

- Maintaining an AIDS-in-the-workplace programme for all education sector employees.

- Making more extensive use of the resources inherent in persons living with HIV/AIDS.

Pay attention to planning, policy and capacity development for HIV/AIDS in education at the national level

Ultimate responsibility for HIV/AIDS and education is national. Regional cooperation can help articulate opportunities and challenges common to many of the countries in the region, but will not be effective unless underpinned by extensive work at the national level. National level work in this area extends to three areas – policy, planning, and capacity development.

The development of policy is crucial. It is essential that the response of an education ministry to HIV/AIDS be guided by a comprehensive policy that extends to the various areas of its responsibility. The policy should cover HIV/AIDS employee issues, such as employment and promotion; testing and confidentiality; counselling, care and support; sexual abuse, substance abuse violence; gender issues; provision of education and training for employees; managing HIV/AIDS in the workplace; conditions of service; and labour relations. For learners, the policy should cover such issues as admission to or continuation in an educational programme; testing and confidentiality; counselling, care and support; rape, sexual abuse, substance abuse, and violence; and gender issues. For the system, the policy should set out the ministry's goals and objectives in dealing with HIV/AIDS in the sector; indicate areas of major intervention (for example, the curriculum); specify the structures that have been established to deal with the epidemic in education; and outline universal general precautions for reducing the risk of HIV transmission in educational institutions.

This book has already given much space to strategic planning for the education sector's response to HIV/AIDS. Such planning is key to a well-considered and effective response. It should be set within the larger framework of a country's national strategic plan for HIV/AIDS (as well as of the Caribbean Regional Strategic Plan of Action). It should be developed in a participatory manner, with the effective involvement of a broad range of partners. It should provide for the structures and processes needed for implementation. It should be implemented, but should also provide for continuous adaptation in response to the changing environment of HIV/AIDS in the sector, country, region and world (for example, in the event of epidemiological changes or of a therapeutic or preventive vaccine becoming available).

Dedicated budgets and capacity are required to drive effective education sector responses to HIV/AIDS. Because the epidemic and its impacts will endure for a very long time, the goal should be to incorporate obligations arising because of HIV/AIDS into core budgets and functions (but with great care that the HIV/AIDS needs and perspectives retain their identity, high profile and urgency). Staff development activities should include training in the skills needed in an education sector that is sensitive to HIV/AIDS and determined to improve the situation. In the appointment of new staff, attention should be given to a good understanding of the interaction between HIV/AIDS and education and to building up the skills needed to manage the impacts in the sector.

Build multisectoral and multilevel partnerships

International, regional and national reports concur in highlighting the key role that strategic alliances, partnerships and collaborative arrangements play in the struggle with HIV/AIDS. In response to an epidemic that enters into so many different facets of life, partnerships are emerging as critical to success. They stretch across the whole of the government sector, with very diverse government ministries and departments working in close cooperation, sometimes for the first time. They are also multilevel, involving government ministries, various organs of civil society, the private sector, and international organisations. At the international level, the central importance of partnerships is given expression in UNAIDS, the joint United Nations programme on HIV/AIDS, which brings together as cosponsors eight United Nations organisations – UNICEF, UNDP, UNFPA, UNDCP, ILO, UNESCO, WHO and the World Bank – each maintaining its own identity, but all cooperating with one another to provide a coordinated response to the many factors driving the HIV epidemic.

Partnerships at regional and national levels are likewise critical to the success of the educator sector's response to HIV/AIDS. The Health and Family Life Education (HFLE) initiative already constitutes an important partnership arrangement, but is restricted largely to curriculum areas. There is room for a broader alliance that embraces the whole range of education's concerns in the context of HIV/AIDS – not merely curriculum, but also teacher development, policy, planning, financing, capacity building, and other areas identified earlier in this book. Such a regional alliance might focus its concerns and activities on the implementation of the 'minimax' principle:

1. minimising the impact of HIV/AIDS on education throughout the region; and

2. maximising the impact of education on HIV/AIDS.

There is also room for the education sector across the region, in its response to HIV/AIDS, to interact in a more structured way both with relevant regional bodies such as the University of the West Indies or the Caribbean Association of Publishers Network (CAPNET), and with the United Nations family and other international agencies (DFID, EU, CIDA, French Aid, etc.). No clear mechanism exists that allows for an approach on the part of the entire Caribbean education sector to regional or international bodies, although it is possible that PANCAP might facilitate this kind of interaction. For the moment, agency support is very varied, lacks coordination, is concerned with detail, and appears not to be guided by any strategic approach (UNESCO Caribbean, 2002). A more structured regional approach, originating from a partnership involving every education sector in the region, would help to identify 'priorities that can best be addressed collectively at a regional level to the benefit of all, while identifying key issues for national level focus that will advance the regional fight against HIV/AIDS' (CRSPAH, 2000: 1).

If a pan-Caribbean educational partnership were established, its success in contributing to the campaign against HIV/AIDS in the region would be determined by the same factors that determine the success of any partnership arrangement. It should be authoritatively established; empowered to take action; trusted by those who have established it; believed in by its members; supported in its operations by the wholehearted collaboration of the various partners; sensitive to the many voices it comprises, the quiet and unobtrusive as much as the strong and compelling; adequately resourced; and accountable for the achievement of results.

Across the region, and within the individual countries, the importance of coalitions with three special civil society partner groups needs to be stressed. Each of them makes an inestimable contribution to HIV/AIDS programmes in the three areas that are of concern to the education sector – HIV prevention, the provision of care and support, and impact mitigation. Synergies arising from collaborative efforts and partnership arrangements between these groups and the educational sector could dramatically affect the progress of the epidemic in the Caribbean. The groups are:

- faith-based organisations;
- youth organisations; and
- women's organisations.

Chapter 7 has already dealt with national level faith-based organisations. Scope exists also at regional level for mutual collaboration with region-wide bodies, such as the Caribbean Council of Churches, the Antilles Episcopal Conference, and regional bodies representing Hindu and Islamic interests. More possibly than many others, these organisations experience intense moral pressure to take the steps needed to overcome the AIDS epidemic. Working in partnership with the education sector in the region, they can take those steps and begin to turn the situation round.

As noted in the opening pages of this book, the opening years of the twenty-first century have been characterised by a new global resolve to tackle HIV/AIDS. Within this framework the need for a particular emphasis on young people has been recognised. 'In every country where HIV transmission has been reduced, it has been among young people (and with their determination) that the most spectacular reductions have occurred' (UNAIDS, 2002a: 16). Young people have always shown willingness to work in partnership with others to overcome HIV/AIDS, but sometimes the world of older people shows more readiness to do things for them than with them. The Caribbean education sector should try to remedy this by providing for strong partnerships with youth organisations, especially in activities that employ peer educators; reach out to young people who are engaged in work which deals with sex, are gay or lesbian, or use drugs; focus on transforming harmful gender stereotypes (macho masculinity and passive femininity); and work against the burdens arising from stigma, discrimination and the strongly homophobic culture that pervades much of the region.

These partnerships should ensure the active participation of young people in the process, and their involvement in the planning and development of preventive and education programmes within the formal education system. The CARICOM Youth Ambassadors programme provides a channel that could make this possible (*Box 24*).

Box 24. The Caribbean Youth Ambassadors in action against HIV/AIDS

The CARICOM Youth Ambassadors initiative seeks to mobilise the talents, energies and resources of young people and channel them into programmes promoting regionalism,

Box 24 (cont'd).

integration and Caribbean unity. The cadre of Ambassadors profile the Caribbean Community model, and promote good citisenship; integrity; peer-bonding (sharing and caring); Caribbean culture and values; and respect for good governance. The philosophy of the Youth Ambassadors is that the youth listen to each other. 'Whether it is hair, fashion, music or sex, the youth speak to each other.' They seek to teach youth to reach youth.

Thus, at a conference held in Surinam in August 2002, a group of youth delegates, meeting under the banner of the Youth Ambassadors, adopted the 'Paramaribo Declaration', urging their government leaders to ensure that youth play a role in telling their peers about HIV/AIDS. The youth also publicly endorsed the regional strategy against HIV/AIDS by signing the 'Pan Caribbean Partnership Commitment', a strategy that focuses on care and treatment for people living with AIDS, prevention and human rights, and reducing stigma. The Youth Ambassadors noted that these three elements all have implications for Caribbean youth who, as a group, are the most highly vulnerable to the disease.

Source: Peter Richards, *Inter Press Service*, September 23, 2002.

The education sector and its other partners should also seek to establish mechanisms that facilitate youth participation at different levels, in formal and non-formal education, and take account of their visions, aspirations and expressed needs. This participation will be enhanced if the education sector and its other partners devote thought and resources to building capacity and strengthening leadership among youth groups. Such investments will reap rich dividends, since youth participation is key to the success of many interventions.

What has been said about the participation of youth applies equally to the involvement of women. Increasingly, women's organisations are focusing on the need to arrest the progress of the epidemic and to offer care, support and treatment to the infected and affected. The education sector can enter into strong alliances with any such groups that may be operating in the Caribbean. As in other parts of the world where women's organisations became systematically involved in the struggle with the epidemic, the outcomes are likely to be beneficial.

Finally, if the education sector is to respond to the HIV/AIDS needs of learners its institutions must be well integrated with the communities they serve. UNAIDS has noted that 'community mobilisation is the core strategy on which success against HIV/AIDS has been built' (UNAIDS, 2002*a*: 16). The crucial responses must occur at community level. To promote responses for young people that work with the community supporting the HIV/AIDS-related activities of the school and the school supporting the HIV/AIDS activities of the community, the gap that often exists between school and community must be bridged (*Chapter 5* above). An important way of doing this is to strengthen the role of school governing boards and parent-teacher associations so that they constitute a more effective link between schools and communities. These bodies can be powerful agents in ensuring appropriate action on HIV/AIDS within the school sector. They can also be very significant in winning community support for school undertakings and in harmonising the approaches and activities of schools and their communities. Strengthening partnerships with them and enhancing their role in the sector's response to the epidemic are essential to the success of that response.

Base the education sector's approach on the three strategies of prevention, care/support, and impact mitigation

The response of the education sector in the Caribbean to HIV/ AIDS should rest on three pillars: prevention of HIV transmission, care and support for those who are infected or affected, and management of the systemic and institutional impacts so as to mitigate their negative effects.

The United Nations has affirmed that 'prevention must be the mainstay of our response' (UNGASS, 2001: 19). Successful prevention reduces the numbers who become infected and eventually results in their tapering off. In recognition of this, and taking account of the high levels of new infections among young people – the principal beneficiaries of educational provision – the United Nations has set 2010 as the target year by which HIV prevalence among young men and women aged 15 to 24 will be reduced by 25 per cent and at least 95 per cent of this age group will have access to the information, education (including peer education and youth-specific HIV education) and services necessary to develop the life skills necessary to reduce their vulnerability to HIV infection (UNGASS, 2001: §47, 53). Much of the responsibility for success in achieving these targets lies with the education sector.

Quantitatively, the education sector in the Caribbean is faced with the responsibility of being a major player in the task of reducing the prevalence rate among young women from 3.2 per cent at the end of 2001 to 2.4 per cent in 2010 and among young men from 2.4 to 1.8 per cent. The Caribbean Regional Strategic Plan of Action has identified the prevention of HIV transmission, with a focus on young people, as one of its six priority areas, and has proposed specific strategic objectives and activities for achieving this goal. The challenge confronting the education sector is to work within the framework of the Regional Plan to further progress in this direction.

There are two important ways in which the education sector can address this challenge. First, it must ensure that every young person in the region can have access to good quality education for as many years as possible. This in itself equips young people with capabilities that support their efforts to keep themselves HIV free. Second, it must establish and provide high quality programmes purposefully directed to HIV prevention so as to equip all learners with the values, attitudes, knowledge and skills that enhance their ability to keep themselves HIV free. By attending to these two areas, the education sector will respond positively to the challenges from the world community and will make a signal contribution to the reduction of HIV prevalence in the Caribbean.

But prevention alone is not a complete response to HIV/AIDS. 'Care, support and treatment are fundamental elements of an effective response' (UNGASS, 2001: 22). In the case of learners, the education sector must make a coherent response to the challenges posed by orphans and those carrying the burdens of abandonment, vulnerability, stigma, shame, poverty and desperation that are all too often experienced when there is AIDS in a family. In the case of educators, the basic need is for the sector to demonstrate its care and concern through its regulations, procedures and systems. These range from those that govern absenteeism and time-off, through those that relate to the workplace, to those concerned with medical schemes, disability, retirement, and death benefits.

An education sector that is characterised by the extent and sensitivity of its care, compassion and support for infected or affected learners, educators and general workforce, is making a powerful and effective response to the epidemic. It is showing through the way it goes about its daily business that there is hope and determination and that HIV/AIDS will not be allowed to conquer.

The third pillar of the sector's response, the creative management of the systemic and institutional impacts of the epidemic on the sector so as to mitigate their negative effects, is equally important. Without attention to this, the system and its institutions could deteriorate to the extent that they would no longer be capable of advancing protection, providing knowledge and understanding, or ensuring care, compassion and support. The system that is meant to protect must itself be protected: 'a critical task will be to protect the core functions of the key social, economic and political institutions, under the onslaught of HIV/AIDS' (UNESCO, 2001: 19).

Attending to these three core dimensions of the education sector's response to the epidemic necessitates commitment to establishing a policy, planning and management framework that will facilitate making and implementing choices about the direction in which the sector must move. The education sector needs to move forward from the rhetoric of notional assent to what is being said about the epidemic to real assent in the form of action. To paraphrase the words of Nelson Mandela when closing the Thirteenth International AIDS Conference in Durban in July 2000, the national and regional education sectors in the Caribbean 'have to rise above their differences and combine their efforts to save their people. History will judge them harshly if they fail to do so – now, and right now'.

Make creative use of the region's rich cultural diversity

HIV/AIDS programming in the Caribbean must make full use of the region's rich cultural diversity for a better understanding of the problem and ways of addressing it. The region is characterised by very different, pervasive and interacting cultures. These include, but are not confined to:

- the more traditional cultures of the peoples of the region – their collective consciousness – with their beliefs, values, customs, standards, languages, idioms, and cultural expressions;

- the parallel Euro-American culture that dominates much economic activity and many life-styles, especially among middle and upper class urban dwellers, and that is fuelled by dynamic interactions with Caribbean communities in North America and Europe and by exposure to the international media;

- the dynamic music culture that expresses the vitality and aspirations of Caribbean peoples, cuts across social and economic boundaries, and has enthused much of the world; and

- the quasi-modern youth culture, with its symbols, expressions, unique role models, the great power of peer pressure, and an almost compulsive need to belong.

A cardinal programming principle is that these cultures should be seen as allies, bringing their own unique resources to the struggle against HIV/AIDS. This has not always been the case. Instead, cultural beliefs and practices have sometimes been characterised as obstacles to be overcome. Efforts to use Caribbean music to carry messages about the epidemic have been criticised on the grounds that they did not come to terms with the realities of the cultures in the region, but were little more than superficial amalgamations of poorly understood AIDS information with even less well understood Caribbean music and culture (Best, 1999). The same may be true of television education-entertainment ('edutainment') soap operas, notwithstanding the potency of these to reach large numbers in an apparently convincing way. In addition, the approaches, thought-patterns, value systems and communication channels used in responding to the epidemic correspond predominantly to the Euro-American perspective and less to the perspectives of local self-understanding, beliefs and practices.

But the principle still remains: HIV/AIDS programming must make creative use of the Caribbean's rich cultural diversity in the struggle against the epidemic. This is a major challenge for education throughout the region. The sector needs to understand how it can better attune its HIV prevention programmes to take account of all the cultural realities (including the very vibrant youth culture) within which these programmes must be embedded. Every aspect of its communication about the epidemic, in schools and in programmes for out-of-school youth, must be sensitive to the codes, meanings, values, beliefs, and assumptions inherent in the common consciousness of the peoples of the Caribbean.

Studies promoted by UNESCO in some Caribbean countries (and also in Southern Africa and South-East Asia) on taking a cultural approach to HIV/AIDS prevention and treatment have revealed extensive misunderstandings about cultural referents and resources and very little attempt to mobilise them for developing relevant protection and care activities (UNESCO/UNAIDS, 2000). The project noted the need for a much better understanding than is currently available of the implications of people's cultural determinants for their responses to the epidemic. For the education sector this has the region's cultural dynamics, with special attention to the implications for the sector's approach to HIV/AIDS, and ensure that educational messages for the Caribbean region take the diverse cultures into account.

Adopt a strong human rights approach

As noted in the opening chapter, a strong human rights approach should guide every response to the HIV/AIDS epidemic. Hence a major strategic thrust of the Caribbean education sector's combat with HIV/ AIDS should be to dedicate resources and efforts to the establishment of an environment in which the practice of human rights can flourish. This will require policies and procedures that fearlessly outlaw every infringement of rights. HIV/AIDS-related issues, which are linked directly to human rights include:

- limitations on the right to education or to a particular type of education because of HIV/AIDS in one's person or one's family;
- HIV/AIDS-related inability to pay for education or for a particular type of education;
- all forms of HIV/AIDS-related stigma and discrimination;
- manifestations of violence and/or sex abuse;
- the exploitation of children or minors;
- gender-based differential treatment;
- interference with the right to seek, receive and impart information and ideas of all kinds (including practical HIV preventive education);
- attacks on honour and reputation;
- denial of the right to facilities for the treatment of illness (including access to youth-friendly health services that can ensure the availability of supplies);
- invasions of privacy and breaches of confidentiality about one's HIV status, sexual orientation or sexual practices.

Positively, systems and their institutions should ensure that their climate is one of acceptance of the HIV/AIDS infected and affected, their practices and procedures demonstrate care and compassion, and their approach is one that sustains hope. A special responsibility at the institutional level is to safeguard provisions for orphans and other children made vulnerable by the epidemic. A further need is to establish links with the social and health services that would ensure the availability of care and support for the infected and affected. Education systems should likewise ensure that their operations are characterised by a caring and compassionate human rights approach. Fundamental to this would be carefully crafted policies, guidelines and regulatory frameworks that are delicately sensitive to the dignity, suffering and anxiety of HIV/AIDS infected and affected learners, teachers and other members of the education workforce.

This revisiting of education within a human rights framework is something that is eminently desirable on its own merits. But the situation of HIV/AIDS accentuates the need for such a review, and more so as the prevalence of the disease increases. While the review needs to be conducted by each country within its own national framework, the outcomes would more clearly constitute an aspect of the education sector's regional response to HIV/AIDS if it were also carried out at regional level, with high level agreement on regional standards and benchmarks.

Make unambiguous provision for the incorporation of gender dimensions

Cultural and behavioural norms affect the course of the HIV/AIDS epidemic in the Caribbean, as they do in other parts of the world. The Regional Plan of Action for HIV/AIDS is stark in the way it presents a number of these:

- Many men and women have multiple sex partners; social and cultural norms condone and even encourage this.

- Poor communication among partners on sexual needs and concerns is coupled with and compounded by women's emotional and socio-economic dependence on men; this limits women's ability to negotiate for safer sex practices.

- There are high levels of sexual violence in some Caribbean societies.

- Widespread use and abuse of alcohol and other substances, especially among young people, often act as disinhibiting factors and facilitate sexual violence and other high-risk behaviours.

- Sexual activity among youth often begins at much earlier ages than is commonly believed by parents, teachers, and other adults.

- Social 'taboos' that prevent teaching or discussing sex with young people deny the incorporation of sex education into school curricula.

- Heavy stigma surrounding same-sex relationships means both individual and societal denial of actual risk.

- Many men who have sex with men also have sexual relationships with women, thereby increasing the risk of HIV transmission to women and children.

- The limited acceptability of condoms restricts their use (CRSPAH: 7).

If the education sector in the region is to be successful in contributing to HIV prevention, it must acknowledge and address these factors in a realistic way. If it fails to do so, it is failing its clients and is failing society.

Gender considerations run through almost all of the adverse behavioural factors enumerated in the Regional Plan. These considerations need to be integrated, frankly and fearlessly, into appropriate education programmes. Three gender-related issues, in particular, appear to warrant the attention of the education sector throughout the region, in terms of the policies and strategies it formulates, the structures and procedures it adopts, and the programmes it teaches – all within the context of HIV/AIDS.

A first and major concern for the education sector is the gender disparity in the region in regard to access to education, school performance and perseverance within the learning environment. In contrast to the situation in the majority of developing countries, the bias within the Caribbean education sector is in favour of girls. Unlike their male counterparts, almost all girls complete the basic primary cycle. Their overall performance surpasses that of boys. More girls than boys proceed to secondary education. At the tertiary level, female students outnumber males several times over and generally outperform males. In many parts of the world, girls are seen as participating in an education system designed for boys. The reverse seems to hold good in the Caribbean: boys participate in an education system that functions as if it were designed for girls.

The lower educational status of boys and young men gives cause for concern throughout the region. As already noted, this is something that the region has to be address within the framework of the EFA goal of the elimination of all gender-based disparities. The region is faced with the major educational challenge of ensuring boys' full and equal access to, and achievement in basic education of good quality. At the same time, it needs to formulate policies and devise strategies that will promote the enrolment of adolescent boys and young men in secondary and tertiary education programmes and that will boost their educational achievement.

The lower educational status of boys and young men is also something that has to be addressed in terms of the implications for HIV/AIDS. Changing economic conditions and the higher levels of education among females seem to be contributing to wider employment and economic participation by females at the expense of males. Confronted with uncertainty about their control over economic resources, males may look for compensation by exercising even more control over females, through unhealthy sexual dominance, multiple partnerships and violence.

> *The erosion of self-esteem and increased materialism in Caribbean societies are key to understanding why Caribbean people continue to expose themselves to risk of HIV through their sexual relationships and behaviours ... Males struggle to maintain their sense of masculinity in the face of economic and symbolic change by maintaining the double*

standard whereby they have multiple partners but women should not. Women fail to protect themselves from HIV because they are more interested in maintaining their femininity by playing the passive sexual role (though their roles in the rest of their lives may be at odds with this) (Allen, 2002: 11).

The education sector across the region can play a crucial role in turning this situation round by more wholehearted dedication in policy and practice to ensuring greater participation and improved performance on the part of boys and young males, that is, it should act dynamically for the eradication of this form of gender disparity in education. The sector should also confront within its programmes, and as appropriate to the level of the learners, the 'machismo' and 'feminismo' images that perpetuate unbalanced sexual practices and relationships. A Jamaican study has called for the establishment of 'a wide-scale public programme targeted at boys and men about alternative conceptions of masculinity and at girls about alternative constructs of femininity' to counter prevalent identity misconceptions (Kempadoo and Dunn, 2002: 217). The entire region would benefit if such a programme were integrated as a matter of principle within the school curriculum as part of HFLE or other suitable area.

The second area of concern is the fragile family structure. 'The family is the natural and fundamental group unit of society and is entitled to protection by society and the State' (Declaration of Human Rights, Article 16 (3)). Within the Caribbean the family needs more of this protection, if only so that young people may grow up with positive parental role models, achieve a better sense of their own sexual identity, and turn with confidence to both male and female care-givers for the guidance, nurturance and support they need. The education sector can enhance the status of the family as the first and vital cell of society by focusing teaching programmes on strengthening family values and using the system to celebrate family. Anything the sector does to boost the role and status of the family will strengthen this social structure in the face of HIV/AIDS, and this in turn can be expected to have a positive knock-on effect on HIV prevention.

A third gender-related area that the education sector in the Caribbean cannot afford to ignore is the strong homophobia that pervades much of the region. Male-to-male sexual contact is a major route for HIV transmission in several countries in the region. In many of these countries, homosexuality is so heavily stigmatised that it has led many individuals to adopt a double way of life, one manifesting overt, visible, socially acceptable heterosexuality, the other concealing covert, secretive, apprehensive homosexuality. This clearly increases the HIV transmission risk for men and women.

Despite the growing numbers of cases in women, attitudes to HIV/ AIDS in many parts of the Caribbean are still rooted in the mistaken perception that it is a man's disease, transmitted primarily through male-to-male sexual contact (Trotman, 1999). This misconception creates a delusion of safety for some who have actually been exposed to the virus, preventing them from facing up to the possibility. It also fuels the stigma and prejudice against HIV-positive heterosexual men and their families. The prevailing homophobia increases the scale of these difficulties. The outcome is an environment that is highly favourable to the effective transmission of HIV.

Because relative ignorance and confusion in the area of human sexuality abound in many parts of the Caribbean, the region would stand to benefit from educational programmes that deal broadly with this subject. This is an urgent need. The programmes must be age-appropriate and the curricula should cover a wide range of topics, including normal sexual development, relationship formation, sex and the law, and sexual diversity. In focusing broadly on human sexuality, young and old learners will grow in their ability to distinguish between consensual sex and situations in which sexual abuse or exploitation occurs, for example, rape and paedophilia. They would also learn to appreciate the root causes of different sexual behaviours and to respect people as individuals rather than ostracising them. Because of the strong homophobia that pervades much of the region, a Caribbean curriculum on human sexuality needs to deal with this topic, showing how homophobic attitudes and practices conflict with those deriving from the perspective of human rights, tolerance, and acceptance of diversity. The education sector can take the lead in developing and implementing such programmes.

Focus on achieving the UNGASS targets

The United Nations has established clear targets for HIV prevention and information among young people aged 15 to 24 and in relation to responding to the needs of orphans and children affected by HIV/AIDS. The attainment of these targets requires purposeful, well planned and properly implemented efforts. They will not just materialise. The central concern of the targets is with young people aged 15 to 24 and orphaned or vulnerable children. The same groups are central within education. Reaching them with the information, skills and support needed for the attainment of the UNGASS targets is a major responsibility of the education sector and a clear direction for its engagement in the coming years. Although the United Nations targets are spelled out in a time-bound fashion, the need for education to be concerned with these areas will persist for several years afterwards, because of the need to consolidate gains, because HIV/AIDS will remain a global problem for decades into the future, and because of the long time-perspective within which the challenge of orphans must be addressed.

The quantitative prevention goals are to reduce HIV prevalence by 25 per cent among those aged 15 to 24 and to ensure that 95 per cent of the same group have access to the information, education and services they need for the development of the life skills that would reduce their vulnerability to HIV, both by 2010 (UNGASS, 2001:§47, 53). An associated qualitative goal is to intensify efforts to challenge gender stereotypes and attitudes and gender inequalities in relation to HIV/AIDS, encouraging the active involvement of men and boys (UNGASS, 2001: §47). All of these have relevance for the education sector.

Other UNGASS HIV concerns are also of relevance for the education system and its programmes:

- establish and implement prevention and care programmes in the work sector (§49);

- ensure the availability of a wide range of prevention programmes that take account of local circumstances, ethics and cultural values (§52);

- ensure information, education and communication aimed at encouraging responsible sexual behaviour, including abstinence and fidelity (§52);

- expand access to condoms and sterile injecting equipment (§52);

- expand access to voluntary counselling and testing and to early and effective treatment of STIs (§52);

- enact, strengthen or reinforce legislation, regulations and other measures to eliminate all forms of discrimination and to ensure the full enjoyment of all human rights and fundamental freedoms by people living with HIV/AIDS and members of vulnerable groups (§58);

- strengthen policies and programmes that recognise the importance of the family in reducing vulnerability (§63);

- ensure the access of both boys and girls to primary and secondary education (§63);

- include HIV/AIDS in the curriculum for adolescents (§63);

- ensure safe and secure environments, especially for young girls (§63);

- expand good-quality, youth-friendly information and sexual health education and counselling services (§63);

- involve young people and families in planning, implementing and evaluating HIV/AIDS prevention and care programmes, as far as possible (§63).

The presentation of these UNGASS concerns gives a broad indication of some directions in which the education sector should be heading in the Caribbean. What will be most problematic for the sector is likely to be the quantitative target of ensuring that almost all 15 to 24 year-olds have access to HIV prevention information, education and services. This is because institutionalised forms of education do not reach everyone in this category. But there are initiatives that the education sector can take throughout the region.

First, it should ensure the inclusion of HIV prevention information and education in every formal programme for young people. Where education ministries have direct control, as they usually do in curriculum materials and teacher development for primary and secondary schools, they should ensure adequate attention to challenging, values-forming, accurate, skills-based HIV-prevention education. This will be accomplished largely through the HFLE initiative, but where appropriate other approaches could be used. Where education ministries do not have direct control, as with many tertiary level training programmes, they should work with the relevant authorities – directly or indirectly through national, regional and international bodies – to ensure that appropriate HIV education and information are incorporated in their programmes. This can be accomplished more readily if partnerships are strong and effective.

Second, education ministries can collaborate with other agencies in the ways advocated in *Chapter 9*, to ensure extensive, coordinated and purposeful HIV prevention education programmes for young people who are not reached by the formal education system. What is important is that the education ministry recognises its responsibility to these individuals and ensures that responding to their needs remains high on its agenda. If other agencies do not speak or act on behalf of the HIV information needs of these young people, the education ministry should be prepared to do so.

Third, the education sector can promote efforts at coordination, information-sharing and networking among those who work in response to the HIV education needs of young people who are outside the formal education system. Programme providers need to be aware of what others are doing in this area and to have some structures for interacting with one another. Education ministries can help in stimulating and supporting such interactions.

Finally, education ministries should examine the progress they are making in attaining the third goal that the world community adopted for itself at the Dakar World Education Forum in 2000, 'ensuring that the learning needs of all young people and adults are met through equitable access to appropriate learning and life-skills programmes' (UNESCO, 2000: 43). The tendency has been to focus on the attainment of universal primary schooling, gender parity in primary and school systems, and quality provision in school education, almost at the expense of what is set forth in this third goal about the broader learning needs of all young people and adults. Renewed attention to these broader learning needs implies attention to HIV learning needs and may be an important route for addressing young people's requirements in this area (*Box 25*).

Box 25. Learning needs of all young people and adults

Better health is a significant trigger for learning. UNICEF has found that programmes designed to prevent and combat HIV/AIDS will be more effective when they are embedded in broad based programmes of social and personal development encompassing generic skills such as communication, negotiation and other interpersonal skills; information gathering, critical thinking and decision making, self-awareness, coping, assertiveness and handling emotions.

Source: UNESCO, *EFA Global Monitoring Report, 2002*: 57.

For orphans, the UNGASS goals include their enrolment in school, their protection from all forms of abuse or violence, and the promotion of an active and visible policy of de-stigmatisation of children orphaned and made vulnerable by HIV/AIDS (UNGASS 2001: §65, 66). Since the challenge presented by the escalating number of orphans to which AIDS is leading has already been dealt with (*Chapter 8*), it will suffice here to reinforce what has already been said by re-affirming some of the programming principles for orphan care. These could well be integrated into a regional strategic framework for the education sector:

- Strengthen the protection and care of orphans and other vulnerable children within their extended families and communities.

- Focus on the most vulnerable children and communities, not only those orphaned by AIDS.

- Ensure the full involvement of young people as part of the solution.

- Strengthen schools and access to education.

- Make specific efforts to address stigma and discrimination.

- Strengthen partners and partnerships at all levels and build coalitions among key stakeholders.

- Ensure that support measures strengthen and do not undermine community initiatives and motivation (UNAIDS/UNICEF/ USAID, 2002: 34-35).

It should be noted that the global Declaration of Commitment on HIV/AIDS included a pledge, on the part of the United Nations General Assembly, to devote at least one full day each year to reviewing progress achieved in realising the agreed-upon goals. To facilitate this ongoing review process, UNAIDS and its partners have developed a set of core indicators that permit monitoring of measurable aspects of the various activities envisaged in the Declaration of Commitment. Countries and regions will use these indicators in reporting back to the United Nations on the progress they are making towards the UNGASS targets (UNAIDS, 2002*b*).

Indicators that are relevant to the education sector are:

- Percentage of schools with teachers who have been trained in lifeskills-based HIV/AIDS education and who taught it during the last academic year.

- Percentage of large enterprises/companies that have HIV/AIDS workplace policies and programmes.

- Percentage of young people aged 15 to 24 who correctly identify ways of preventing the sexual transmission of HIV and who reject major misconceptions about HIV transmission.
- Ratio of current school attendance among orphans to that among non-orphans, aged 10 to 14 (UNAIDS, 2002a: 23).

Strengthen the sector's ability to develop the ideal Caribbean person

Almost all of the qualities sketched by the CARICOM Heads of State in their profile of the 'ideal Caribbean person' are antithetical to HIV/AIDS – respect for human life, emotional security, being comfortable with differences, responsible, accountable to family and community, secure in cultural identity (*Box 26*). A person endowed with these qualities is not likely to engage in behaviour that risks HIV infection or transmission, will not resort to stigma or discrimination, is likely to manifest compassion and care, and is equipped to counteract the adverse socioeconomic impacts of the epidemic.

Box 26. Qualities of the ideal Caribbean person

The ideal Caribbean person:

- Respects human life as the foundation on which all of the other desired values must rest.
- Is emotionally secure.
- Values differences based on gender, ethnicity, religion and other forms of diversity as sources of strength and richness.
- Is environmentally aware.
- Is responsible and accountable to family and community.
- Has a strong work ethic.
- Is creative and entrepreneurial.
- Has an informed respect for the cultural heritage.

Source: Jules and Panneflek, 2000: 63.

The Heads of Government also saw education as playing a critical role in the development of this holistic Caribbean person (Jules and Panneflek, 2000: 63). The more whole-hearted adoption by the education sector of this vision, and its embodiment in policies, procedures and curriculum, would be a significant stride forward in the use of education to counteract HIV/AIDS. Through the further affirmation of this vision in the context of HIV/AIDS, education authorities in the Caribbean would signal that education's ideal is about:

- Respecting life, and hence working against every possibility of HIV transmission and excluding all forms of violence.

- Becoming emotionally secure, and hence fostering the development of a mature personal sexuality, understanding of relationship and self-possessed acceptance of one's sexual identity.

- Valuing differences in others as sources of strength, and hence accepting persons living with HIV/AIDS, those from families where there is HIV/AIDS, and persons with different sexual orientations, as fellow human beings to be respected and valued in themselves and for the new understandings they can bring to human problems.

- Becoming environmentally aware, and hence recognising the role of good environmental conditions, safe water and sanitation, and good nutrition in the preservation of health and strengthening against HIV infection.

- Developing in responsibility and accountability, and hence taking every possible measure to strengthen the family and ensure that HIV is not introduced into the family or community, and should AIDS have brought sickness or death, ensuring care with dignity for the sick and support with humanity for orphans.

- Growing in the spirit of conscientiousness, work and industry, and hence not having recourse to the sale of sex or traffic in drugs for self-support or personal advancement.

- Developing a creative, entrepreneurial spirit, and hence seeing a great need to protect the future and not to jeopardise it through drug use, alcohol abuse or taking the risk of HIV infection.

- Increasing in the knowledge, love and experience of the cultural heritage, and hence celebrating life and protecting it from the destructive effects of HIV, drug use and alcohol abuse.

In other words, this truly Caribbean-originated and owned vision of the ideal Caribbean person could mark out major directions that would guide the education sector across the region in confronting and getting the better of HIV/AIDS.

AFTERWORD
Opportunity in Crisis

An epidemic is most often described as a dynamic progression, in which an infection jumps from one person to another in a population, and where the risk of contracting it is a function of both the number already infected and those not yet infected. In graphical terms the process can often be depicted as an S-shaped curve – slow at first, then accelerating, and then spreading more slowly as people learn to take precautions and fewer are left to become infected.

But this book also tells a different story. It shows how an epidemic can be embedded in the very social make-up of a society. The way it spreads and whom it affects is shaped by the institutional arrangements of the society concerned: structure influences dynamics and social organisation shapes the flow of events.

A simple illustration of this thesis is found in the widely differing rates of the spread of the HIV/AIDS epidemic in Western and non-Western societies. In many of the former, after the early leap in cases, the rate of new infections has to a large extent flattened out. The rise in the S did not go very far, though there have been notable setbacks, for example in the USA where the number of new HIV/ AIDS cases rose in 2002 for the first time in a decade. In countries like Australia or Norway, the reactions to the epidemic were swift, comprehensive and resolute – and their impacts were immediate, substantial and durable. The strategies used ranged along the scale from public information and non-discrimination, to the provision of treatments. This book tells a similar story for the Caribbean countries – the outstanding case of Cuba reflects its institutional arrangements as well as political response, parts of which have been controversial.

The same has been observed in some developing countries, like Uganda, that have faced similar problems on a much greater scale.

This observation provides us with perhaps the most interesting and optimistic fact about HIV/AIDS – that it is within human capability to curb the spread of the epidemic. But the most paradoxical fact is that this, the most devastating of all epidemics, is caused by a generally avoidable infection. At the same time, the longer the delay in appropriate response, the more costly and difficult it becomes to match the reach of the virus and equal its manifold devastations with adequate measures.

This structural perspective on the epidemic can also be put in other terms. In order to figure out the functioning of a system, it has to be given some stimulus. From the reactions of the system to the stimulus, we can map its inner workings.

HIV/AIDS provides a severe jolt to any society. From the response of the society to the epidemic, we can learn how it is constructed and how it functions. The HIV/AIDS epidemic highlights the social structure through which it spreads. However, there is a very important difference between a social system and other systems. A social system can learn, from understanding, what happens and what works in order to modify itself.

This gives an additional reason for optimism: any social system can be self-correcting – it can learn not just from its own past but also from the experiences of others. The first part of this book provides us with a rich set of opportunities for learning. For example, though HIV/AIDS does not respect social barriers, poverty facilitates its transmission and accelerates the transformation of HIV infection into full-blown AIDS. The lower the level of education, the higher the risk of infection. The harsher the discrimination of the infected and affected, the better the conditions for further spread of the virus. The weaker the position of one sex, the stronger the impact of the epidemic.

In the case of the Commonwealth Caribbean, we see the phenomenon of male *marginalisation*, whereby girls make up the majority of enrolments in, and graduates from secondary schools. Women predominate in most middle class professions, although men often have the most prominent positions in politics and private firms. From such observations policy implications can be drawn.

The HIV/AIDS epidemic is an unparalleled development disaster. Its impacts are already more devastating than any war. It attacks not just human bodies, but the body politic as well, with unequalled institutional impact. It undermines the organisations most needed for development, as well as those most needed for curbing the epidemic itself. It erodes access to education, interferes with the capacity of key institutions to function, and in some countries governance itself may be threatened. Children are at risk on an unparalleled scale: millions are orphaned and infected and will grow up deprived and disconnected (UNESCO, 2001).

The epidemic also attacks the very heart of global concerns. The epidemic knows no frontiers and undermines all aspects of sustainable development – reducing poverty, advancing equity, improving health, enhancing human rights and securing education for all. The high rate of disease and death among teachers, health workers and other professionals and also workers trained in particular skills, such as farmers or miners, reduces family incomes and diverts family resources to cover increasing medical costs. Indeed, the epidemic undermines whole economies. As stated in UNESCO's *Strategy for HIV/AIDS preventive education*:

> HIV/AIDS is the deadly nexus between all the items on the world development agenda. It increases inequalities between the different regions of the world, and widens the gap between the rich and the poor (UNESCO, 2001).

The epidemic steals from human development and wipes out decades of investment in education. It creates severe loss of breadwinners, heads of households, professionals and resources and leads to a growth in the number of orphans. This factor makes fighting the epidemic more taxing.

Lack of explicit confrontation and openness may harden prejudice. It undermines the institutions most needed for development – as well as those most needed for curbing the epidemic itself. So the causes are bi-directional – the effects of the epidemic often exacerbate it, as when orphaned children go without education, they grow up poorer and more vulnerable. In short: the circles are multiple, interlocking and vicious.

It is this dynamic complexity of the epidemic that negates the possibility of treating it as just a health problem. The HIV/AIDS epidemic not only highlights all aspects of the social structure in a country: mindsets, attitudes, institutions, economy, etc, but it interacts with all these aspects. Hence it must be confronted in many different ways. Like a carpet that cannot be lifted at only one corner, the HIV/AIDS epidemic cannot be offset by actions from only one angle. A multisectoral and a multifaceted response are needed.

All the more so as there is no cure. No vaccine is in sight. Treatments that can make an otherwise deadly infection into a chronic, yet manageable disease, are too costly and still beyond reach for most of those infected. The epidemic is not levelling off and it is becoming truly global in its reach.

But this need not make us dejected or defeatist. The immensity of the epidemic means that it cannot be ignored or met with complacency. And that is a cause for optimism.

Multi-faceted responses are now being more sharply defined. The Declaration of Commitment on HIV/AIDS of the United Nations General Assembly Special Session in June 2001 is a good illustration. *More resources are being mobilised* – the Global Fund to Fight AIDS, Tuberculosis and Malaria is a case in point. By summer 2003, the Global Fund had attracted US$ 4.7 billion in pledges over 8 years from 40 countries, major foundations (such as the Gates Foundation) and private donors. To mount an effective global response, it has been estimated that some US$ 10 billion a year must be raised by 2005. Much of it will have to come from the affected countries themselves, but the Global Fund will certainly channel a significant amount. And more capacity is being marshalled – the efforts of the Joint United Nations programme on AIDS – UNAIDS – its Secretariat and Cosponsors (WHO, World Bank, UNESCO, UNICEF, UNDP, UNFPA, ILO, UNDCP), national governments as well as NGOs, is a prominent example. The more extensive and better-organised the response, the more reason there is for optimism – even if the response is far behind and far too small.

Another important reason for optimism is that the response can be no single-point programme and no single-actor affair. This means that unsustainable social arrangements and untenable modes of behaviour will cave in. It could be called 'the Frank Sinatra law of social change': "Something's gotta give".

This has happened in former periods of great social crisis. During the First and Second World Wars, for example, women were mobilised for jobs from which they had formerly been excluded – behaviour changed and attitudes followed.

The same is bound to happen as a consequence of the HIV/AIDS epidemic. There is no way of stopping the epidemic if gender inequalities persist, if the greater part of the young remains uneducated, if poverty endures or if discrimination against the infected and affected is not banished. Kofi Annan put it another way: 'All cultures will be pushed to put cultural mores aside to save lives.' (*New York Times*, June 21, 2001).

Hence the present crisis has a hidden potential: it is not just a danger, it is a devastation, yet it is a portent of opportunities that is already here, for constructive change.

The crisis forces us – urgently – to do what we have been advocating for a long time but in fact have continually postponed. We have said we would invest more in education for all. We have said we would deal with gender inequities. We have said we would eradicate poverty. We have said we would advance human rights. Now the cost of not doing it can be counted not only in dollars and dimes, but also in lives lost and communities devastated. And procrastination not only means added loss but also a multiplication of what it will take to measure up to the challenge – the epidemic does not wait. The epidemic has already pushed us beyond the point of no return. The only question that remains is how much we could lose before we act on a small scale and how much worse we will let it become before we respond in full.

The first part of the job of responding to the epidemic is to describe the situation we are in and the predicament we face in open, truthful, and indeed stark language. Furthermore, the response should not only make us grasp the magnitude but also make us understand with our heart and imagination the desperate human dimensions of the problems. Reading this book has had that effect. More information is needed at the global and at the local level. It is not just about the health aspects of the epidemic, but also about the social aspects – about the practices and attitudes that need to change. This book provides us with information – but equally important, with inspiration as well.

The second function is to identify the causes at the root of the present problems. On the one hand, analysis of social meanings and causes can identify unsustainable activities, on the other it can help imagine sustainable alternatives and devise strategies for educating and empowering whole communities. To take one example from the book: confidentiality is a must if people are to test for their HIV status. But in small island communities with close and warm interactions to sustain them, this is hard to ensure because health care workers know and are on close terms with everybody. Hence, there is constant fear of disclosure and being cut off if one is HIV positive.

The third part of the undertaking, therefore, is to provide proposals for new initiatives and policies. Throughout this book there are many of those, ranging the introduction of strategic planning in the education sector to concrete measures for caring for orphans and reaching out to school youth. These proposals come with a value added because they suggest that taking these initiatives will not only help curb and alleviate the epidemic, but will see improvements in the overall quality and relevance of education, indeed, in the whole functioning of communities as well. The proposals are eminently practical and concrete – yet as an ensemble are comprehensive and can be momentous.

More generally, there are very attractive opportunities for general social improvements triggered by efforts to respond to the AIDS crisis in education. In a way, the epidemic can make us more imaginative and effective in whom we educate and how we educate, than we would be in its absence. To illustrate this:

- Education, not least in developing countries, is in a sense a prisoner of its past – often its colonial past – with excessive stress and status being given to academic training. The epidemic directs us to a rethinking of the primary school curriculum, making it more practical and relevant to community and real world needs, in response to society's need for skills replenishment in the context of AIDS, and to the needs experienced by orphans and many young children who will have to enter the world of work immediately after leaving school (and sometimes to take up work while still at school). In short, the curriculum should fall more in line with UNESCO's (1996) 'learning to do' concept – and hence accelerate reforms that are desirable in themselves. In this case necessity can be, if not the mother, at least the midwife of invention.

- Redefining the goals of education to include AIDS competence on the part of every school leaver has implications for the ability to manage oneself and one's relationships. This points in the direction of UNESCO's pillar of 'learning to be', education seeking to promote the integral, harmonious development of the intellectual, affective, moral and spiritual endowments of all students so that they can develop into complete, autonomous and compassionate persons.

- There needs to be a more extensive school-wide concern with 'learning to live together' and a human rights approach, in view of the problems brought by HIV/AIDS stigma, discrimination and the secrecy that surrounds the disease and facilitates its transmission. HIV/AIDS provides a pedagogical opportunity as well as a social necessity of the 'recognition of the inherent dignity and of the equal and inalienable rights of all members of the human family', as is stated in the preamble to the Universal Declaration of Human Rights.

- The local community, with its natural environment and its economic activity, is itself a vital part of the school's learning environment. In the communitarian approach, the community shares some of the responsibilities of individual behaviour, and hence carries a certain collective responsibility to avoid HIV transmission. To this end, it is necessary to narrow the gap between school and community to ensure coherence between the HIV/AIDS messages being communicated in the two settings. Schools are well situated to serve as community resources and can assist in all its development efforts (health, welfare, agriculture, etc.) thereby transcending boundaries between sectors so that development is directed towards individuals and families in their totality. Addressing HIV/AIDS can become an effective way of achieving this broader and often neglected goal. This in turn can lead to much closer links than in the past between schools and their communities, thus enriching the more formal curriculum. Greater parental involvement in the design of school programmes, initiated by the need to secure parental and community approval for the HIV/AIDS and sexuality components of the curriculum is related to this.

- This goal could be further deepened by developing the 'integrated teacher' approach (described in the book and now being adopted in Cuba). With the integrated teacher approach, classes up to the end of lower secondary school, receive all of their instruction from one teacher (apart from one or two very specialised subjects). The teacher's thorough knowledge of the members of the class would be supplemented by regular interaction with the principal family members, so that he or she could develop a thorough, all-embracing, mentoring relationship with the students, families and the community. He or she would be a respected and close authority figure that young people need in the circumstances of HIV/AIDS. The teacher develops multifaceted relations with the students and can have close and multiple relations with parents.

- In this book it is argued and demonstrated that education means protection from HIV/AIDS. The more you get, the better you are protected, which proves you cannot fight HIV/

AIDS without promoting and protecting education – an additional argument for the commitment to Education for All. Knowledge about HIV, what it is, how it is transmitted and how one can protect oneself against it is a key task for schools, yet preventive education cannot be restricted to them as so many children are out of school. And this is a proportion that increases with age. The partial and often faulty information youth receive from peers has to be countered by effective non-formal education. In the context of AIDS, preventive education is too important to be left to schools alone. Schools do not reach all and they reach fewer in the age groups most at risk (UNESCO, 2001). The urgency of extending education programmes to out-of-school youth is in line with UNESCO's life-long learning approach and the third goal of the Dakar Framework for Action to provide education for all. It ensures that 'the learning needs of all young people and adults are met through equitable access to appropriate learning and life-skills programs', since these are the critical population groups within which levels of HIV infection must be reduced.

The potential of a new coalition of school and community shows that while it is true that the epidemic is embedded in countries and communities, it is also true that there are opportunities embedded in the epidemic. Instead of the epidemic causing us to lose control and community, we should try to convert the crisis and recast the tragedy into profound changes long desired – for education, for human rights and for compassion.

We must therefore not only recognise the dangers, but also identify the opportunities inherent in the epidemic. Rather than letting it result in a fatalistic slide towards institutional collapse, we can take it as a break for deliberate remodelling of our societies and a remaking of our social relations – for breakthrough rather than breakdown. Together we need to identify the many benefits that can flow from addressing our common calamity – benefits in more humane and more effective policies to achieve what we have long stated as our goals and follow up by setting in motion the many small projects that can make the big difference.

In this way we can turn our perspective from despair and inaction to confidence and ingenuity. What is more, we can turn the tide.

Gudmund Hernes
Director, IIEP, UNESCO HIV/AIDS Coordinator

REFERENCES

A portrait of adolescent health in the Caribbean. 2000. Minnesota: WHO Collaborating Centre on Adolescent Health, University of Minnesota; Barbados: Caribbean Program Coordination Office of the Pan-American Health Organization/World Health Organization.

Ainsworth, M.; Filmer, D. "Poverty, AIDS and children's schooling: a targeting dilemma". In: *World Bank Policy Research Working Paper* 2885. September 2002. Washington, DC: World Bank, Operations Evaluation Department and Development Research Group.

Allen, C.F. 2002. "Gender and the transmission of HIV in the Caribbean". In: S. Courtman (Ed.), *The Society for Caribbean Studies Annual Conference Papers, 3.*

An ILO code of practice on HIV/AIDS and the world of work. 2001. Geneva: International Labour Office (ILO).

Badcock-Walters, P. 2002. "Education". In: J. Gow and C. Desmond (Eds.), *Impacts and interventions. The HIV/AIDS epidemic and the children of South Africa.* Pietermaritzburg: University of Natal Press.

Barnett, T.; Whiteside, A. 2002. *AIDS in the twenty-first century.* Basingstoke: Palgrave MacMillan.

Bennell, P.; Hyde, K.; Swainson, N. 2002. *The impact of the HIV/AIDS epidemic on the education sector in sub-Saharan Africa. A synthesis of the findings and recommendations of three country studies.* Brighton: Centre for International Education, University of Sussex Institute of Education.

Best, C. 2000. "Caribbean music and the discourse on AIDS". In: G. Howe and A. Cobley (Eds.), *The Caribbean AIDS epidemic.* Kingston: University of the West Indies Press.

Bain, B. and Morrissey, M. 2002. *The Caribbean HIV/AIDS epidemic:* 14-point proposal for *priority curriculum and programming responses by UWI.* Kingston: UWI HARP, University of the West Indies, Mona Campus.

Braslavsky, C. 2002. "Scaling up the response to HIV/AIDS within education systems". In: *Prospects*, 32(2), 3-4.

Centers for Disease Control and Prevention. 2003. *CDC HIV/STD/ TB prevention news update*, 7 January 2003.

Commonwealth universities in the age of HIV/AIDS. *Guidelines towards a strategic response and good practice*. 2002. London: ACU, April 2002.

Coombe, C; Kelly, M. J. 2001. "Education as a vehicle for combating HIV/ AIDS". *Prospects*, 31(3), 435-445.

Crewe, M. 2000. "HIV/AIDS and the University of Pretoria. Implications for the University of Namibia". In: B. Otaala (Ed.), *HIV/AIDS: The challenge for tertiary institutions in Namibia*. Proceedings of a Workshop, 9-11 October 2000. Windhoek, Namibia.

Dicks, B. (Ed.) 2001. *HIV/AIDS and children in the English Speaking Caribbean*. New York: The Haworth Press.

Donovan, P. 2000. *The Impact of HIV and AIDS on the rights of the child to education; discrimination and HIV/AIDS-related stigma and access to education – the response*. Paper presented at SADC-EU Seminar on the Rights of the Child in a World with HIV and AIDS, Harare, Zimbabwe, 23 October, 2000.

Dunn, L.L. 2002. "Promoting adolescent participation in Jamaica". In: *Meeting adolescent development and participation rights. The findings of five research studies on adolescents in Jamaica*. Kingston: UNICEF; UNFPA.

Eberstadt, N. 2002. "The future of AIDS". In: *Foreign Affairs*, 81(6), 22-45.

Engagement as a core value for the university: a consultation document. 2001. London: ACU.

Feachem, R. 2003. Interview reported in Global Fund Observer (GFO) *Newsletter, A service of Aidspan*, 2, 10 January 2003.

Francis, C.R. 2000. "The psychosocial dynamics of the AIDS epidemic in the Caribbean". In: G. Howe and A. Cobley (Eds.), *The Caribbean AIDS epidemic*. Kingston: University of the West Indies Press.

Gachuhi, D. 1999. *The impact of HIV/AIDS on education systems in the eastern and Southern Africa region and the response of education systems to HIV/AIDS: Life skills* programmes. Paper presented to the All Sub-Saharan Africa Conference on Education for All 2000, Johannesburg, December 1999.

Gordon, D.F. 2002. The next wave of HIV/AIDS: *Nigeria, Ethiopia, Russia, India and* China. ICA 2002-04D. September 2002. Washington, DC: National Intelligence Council.

Hawes, H; Stephens, D. 1990. *Questions of quality. Primary education and development.* Harlow: Longman.

Heap, B.; Simpson, A. 2002. *Future positive: educating Zambian children in a time of HIV/AIDS through process drama.* A report for Save the Children, Sweden, June, 2002.

Hernes, G. 2002. "UNESCO versus AIDS: the history and ten lessons". In: *Prospects*, 32(2), 5-11.

Howe, G; Cobley, A. (Eds.). 2000. *The Caribbean AIDS epidemic.* Kingston: University of West Indies Press.

IATT (Inter Agency Task Team on Education). 2002. *HIV/AIDS and education. A strategic approach.* October, 2002. New York: UNICEF.

IBE (International Bureau of Education). 1999. *Survey on curriculum development needs at the upper primary and secondary education levels in the Caribbean sub-region.* Retrieved in May, 1999 from http://www.ibe.unesco.org/Regional/CaribbeanSur vey/caribbee.htm.

Jackson, H. 2002. *AIDS Africa. Continent in crisis.* SAfAIDS: Harare.

Impacts of HIV/AIDS on the South African Departments of Education. 2001. Technical report submitted to the Department of Education. Johannesburg: ABT Associates South Africa.

Jules, V.; Panneflek, A. 2000. *Lighting the way forward. Sub-regional summary and action plan. EFA in the Caribbean*: Assessment 2000. Sub-Regional Report, 1. Kingston: UNESCO.

Kelly, M. J. 2000. "Standing education on its head: aspects of schooling in a world with HIV/AIDS". In: *Current Issues in Comparative Education (CICE)*, 3(1). New York: Teachers' College Columbia. Retrieved from www.tc.columbia.edu/cice.

Kempadoo, K; Dunn, L.L. 2002. "Factors that shape the initiation of early sexual activity among adolescent boys and girls". In: *Meeting adolescent development and participation rights. The findings of five research studies on adolescents in Jamaica.* Kingston: UNICEF; UNFPA.

Kiragu, K. 2001. Youth and HIV/AIDS: *Can we avoid catastrophe?* Population Reports, Series L, No. 12. Population Information Program, Bloomberg School of Public Health. Baltimore: Johns Hopkins University.

Liebowitz, J. 2002. *The impact of faith-based organizations on HIV/ AIDS prevention and mitigation in Africa.* Paper prepared for the Health Economics and AIDS Research Division (HEARD), University of Natal, Durban, South Africa, October 2002.

Longman. 2000. *Longman Caribbean school atlas for social studies, geography and history.* San Juan, Trinidad: Lexicon Trinidad.

Meeks Gardner, J; Powell, C; Grantham-McGregor, S. 2001. *A case-control study of family and school determinants of aggression in Jamaican children.* Kingston: Planning Institute of Jamaica.

Miller, P. 2001. *The lesser evil: the catholic church and the AIDS epidemic.* Washington, DC: Catholics for a Free Choice.

Ministère de l'Education Nationale de la Jeunesse et des Sports (MENJS), Haiti. 2002. *Plan stratégique sectoriel de l'éducation pour la prévention et la lutte contre le VIH/SIDA.* Port au Prince: MENJS.

Ministry of Education, Swaziland. 1999. *Impact Assessment of HIV/AIDS on the Education Sector.* Mbabane: Ministry of Education.

Morrissey, M. 2002. *Should Caribbean publishers contribute textbooks to the fight against the HIV/AIDS epidemic?* Discussion Paper. Findings of an informal survey for UWI HARP, University of the West Indies, Kingston.

Mugabe, M.; Stirling, M.; Whiteside, A. 2002. *Future imperfect: protecting children on the brink.* Discussion paper presented to Africa Leadership Consultation: Acting for children on the brink. Johannesburg, 10 September 2002.

Piot, P. 2000. In: *World education forum, Dakar, Final Report*, 22. Paris: UNESCO.

Report on the national youth KABP survey on HIV/AIDS. 2001. St. Michael, Barbados: Division of Youth Affairs.

Robinson, J. 2002. *Preparing for the vibes in the world of sexuality: Facilitator's manual and activities workbook* (Revised edition for schools). Kingston, Jamaica: Ashe Caribbean Performing Foundation.

Robinson, J. 2002. *Parenting vibes in the world of sexuality: Facilitator's manual.* Kingston, Jamaica: Ashe Caribbean Performing Foundation.

Schenker, I. 2001. *Production, development and implementation of pedagogical approaches and methods for HIV/AIDS prevention in schools.* Presentation to Senior Expert Conference on HIV/AIDS and Education in ECOWAS Countries, Elmina, Ghana, 19-24 March, 2001.

Schenker, I.I.; Nyirenda, J.M. 2002. *Preventing HIV/AIDS in schools.* IBE Educational Practices Series 9. Geneva: International Bureau of Education (IBE).

Stillwaggon, E. 2000. "HIV/AIDS in Africa: fertile terrain". In: *South African Journal of Economics*, 68(5).

Strengthening the institutional response to HIV/AIDS/STI in the Caribbean (SIRHASC). Implementing Document to Framework Financing Agreement No. 6054/REG. 2000. Brussels: European Commission, Directorate-General VIII, Development.

Stuart, W.T.; Bain, B.C. 1993. "Risk factors and behaviour change in HIV-positive women in Nassau, Bahamas. A case control study". In: *West Indies Medical Journal*, 42, Suppl. 1, 34-35.

The Caribbean Regional Strategic Plan of Action for HIV/AIDS. 2000. Caribbean Task Force on HIV/AIDS.

Theodore, K. 2000. *HIV/AIDS in the Caribbean: Economic issues – impact and investment response.* Discussion Paper. Kingston: University of the West Indies.

Trotman, L. 2000. "HIV/AIDS in the workplace. The workers' perspective". In: G. Howe and A. Cobley (Eds.), *The Caribbean AIDS epidemic.* Kingston: University of the West Indies Press.

United Nations. 1998. *HIV/AIDS and Human Rights. International Guidelines.* New York: United Nations.

United Nations, 2002. *HIV/AIDS and Human Rights. Guideline 6.* New York: United Nations.

UNAIDS. 1997. *Impact of HIV and sexual health education on the sexual behaviour of young people: a review update.* Geneva: UNAIDS.

UNAIDS. 1998a. *Guide to the strategic planning process for a national response to HIV/AIDS.* Geneva: UNAIDS.

UNAIDS. 1998b. *AIDS epidemic update: December 1998.* Geneva: UNAIDS.

UNAIDS. 1999a. *World AIDS campaign with children and young people. Key issues and ideas for action.* Geneva: UNAIDS.

UNAIDS. 1999b. *Communications framework for HIV/AIDS. A new direction. A UNAIDS/Penn State Project.* Geneva: UNAIDS.

UNAIDS. 2000a. *Men and AIDS – a gendered approach.* Geneva: UNAIDS, March 2000.

UNAIDS. 2000b. *Report on the global HIV/AIDS epidemic, June 2000.* Geneva: UNAIDS.

UNAIDS. 2001. *AIDS epidemic update: December 2001.* Geneva: UNAIDS.

UNAIDS. 2002a. *Report on the global HIV/AIDS epidemic, July 2002.* Geneva: UNAIDS.

UNAIDS. 2002b. *Implementation of the Declaration of Commitment on HIV/AIDS: core indicators.* Geneva: UNAIDS.

UNAIDS. 2002c. *AIDS epidemic update*. December 2002. Geneva: UNAIDS.

UNAIDS/UNICEF/USAID. 2002. *Children on the brink 2002. A joint report on orphan estimates and program strategies*. Washington, DC: TvT Associates.

UNAIDS/UNICEF/WHO. 2002. *Young people and HIV/AIDS. Opportunity in crisis*. Geneva: UNAIDS; New York: UNICEF; Geneva: WHO.

UNDP. 2001. *Human Development Report 1999*. New York: UNDP.

UNECA. 2000. *HIV/AIDS and education in eastern and southern Africa. The leadership challenge and the way forward*. Synthesis Report for Africa Development Forum 2, October 2000. Addis Ababa: United Nations Economic Commission for Africa (UNECA).

UNESCO. 1996. *Learning. The treasure within (The Delors Report). Report to UNESCO of the International Commission on Education for the Twenty-First Century*. Paris: UNESCO.

UNESCO. 2000. *World Education Forum, Dakar. Final Report*. Paris: UNESCO.

UNESCO. 2001. *UNESCO's strategy for HIV/AIDS preventive education*. Paris: IIEP-UNESCO.

UNESCO. 2002. *Education for All. Is the world on track? EFA global monitoring report 2002*. Paris: UNESCO.

UNESCO Caribbean. 2002. *United Nations support for HIV/AIDS prevention and mitigation in the Caribbean through the Education sector*. Kingston: UNESCO Office for the Caribbean.

UNESCO/UNAIDS. 2000. *A cultural approach to HIV/AIDS prevention and care. Summary of country assessments and project design handbook*. Studies and Reports Series, No. 10, Cultural Policies for Development Unit. Paris: UNESCO.

UNGASS. 2001. *Declaration of Commitment on HIV/AIDS*. United Nations General Assembly, 26th Special Session, 27 June 2001. New York: United Nations.

UNICEF. 2000. *The progress of nations, 2000*. New York: UNICEF.

UNICEF. 2002. *The state of the world's children 2003*. New York: UNICEF.

UNICEF/UNFPA. 2002. *Meeting adolescent development and participation rights. The findings of five research studies on adolescents in Jamaica*. Kingston: UNICEF; UNFPA.

UNICEF/UNFPA. 2002. *Meeting adolescent development and participation rights. The findings of five research studies on adolescents in Jamaica.* Kingston: Jamaica Coalition on the Rights of the Child.

UWI HARP. 2002. UWI HARP Strategic Planning Workshop, University of the West Indies, Mona, 7-8 August, 2002.

Vandemoortele, J.; Delamonica, E. 2000. "The 'education vaccine' against HIV". In: *Current Issues in Comparative Education* (Teachers' College, Columbia University, New York), 3(1). Online version: www.tc.columbia.edu/cice.

Voison, D.R.; Dillon-Remy, M. 2001. "Psychocultural factors associated with HIV infection among Trinidad and Tobago adolescents". In: B.A. Dicks (Ed.), *HIV/AIDS and children in the English speaking Caribbean.* New York: The Haworth Press.

Walrond, E.R. 2000. "Regional policies in relation to the HIV/AIDS epidemic in the Commonwealth Caribbean". In: G. Howe; A. Cobley (Eds.), *The Caribbean AIDS epidemic.* Kingston: University of West Indies Press.

Weindling, D. 1997. "Strategic planning in schools: some practical techniques". In: M. Preedy, R. Glatter, R. Levacic (Eds.), *Educational management: strategy, quality and resources.* Buckingham: Open University Press.

Whiteside, A.; Sunter, C. 2000. AIDS: *The challenge for South Africa.* Cape Town: Human & Rousseau; Tafelberg.

Williams, L. 2002. "Adolescence and violence in Jamaica". In: *Meeting adolescent development and participation rights. The findings of five research studies on adolescents in Jamaica.* Kingston: UNICEF; UNFPA.

World Bank. 2000. *HIV/AIDS in the Caribbean: issues and options. A background report.* Washington, DC: World Bank, Human Development Sector Management Unit, Latin America and the Caribbean Region.

World Bank. 2002. *Education and HIV/AIDS: a window of hope.* Washington, DC: World Bank.

World Bank. 2003. *Education and HIV/AIDS: a sourcebook of HIV/ AIDS prevention programmes.* Washington, DC: World Bank.

APPENDIX I

Havana Commitment of Caribbean Ministers of Education

We, Ministers of Education in the Caribbean, in the context of the Regional Meeting of Ministers of Education of Latin America and the Caribbean (MINEDLAC), November 14-16, 2002, recognising the potential of HIV/AIDS to deplete the human resources needed for sustainable development in the Caribbean, reassert the determination of our Governments to fight the epidemic.

We recognise that Education is integral to the fight against AIDS, and that the disease will not be overcome without the full involvement of the education sector.

We further recognise the need to work in close harmony with other sectors in our countries, and for a regional approach in the framework of the Pan Caribbean Partnership Against Aids.

In this light:

- we acknowledge that more could be done through the education of teachers and students to prevent the spread of HIV;
- we affirm that there is need to provide support and care to affected educators and learners;
- we recognise that creative measures are needed to reduce the impact of the epidemic on our education sectors.

Moved by these and similar considerations, we request UNESCO to assist the Pan Caribbean Partnership Against Aids to establish a regional forum on HIV/AIDS and Education.

We commit ourselves and our Ministries of Education to a heightened and concerted response to HIV/AIDS, beginning from this moment and continuing until, through education and other means, we have entered a world without AIDS.

Havana, CUBA
November 15, 2002

The following Ministers signed the Commitment in Havana, on November 15, 2002, or subsequently.

- The Hon. Rodney Williams
  Minister of Education & Culture
  Antigua & Barbuda

- The Hon. Alfred M. Sears
  Attorney General & Minister of Education
  The Commonwealth of Bahamas

- The Hon. Rudolph Greenidge
  Minister of Education, Youth Affairs & Sports
  Barbados

- The Hon. Francis W. Fonseca
  Minister, Education, Youth & Sports
  Office of the Prime Minister, Belize

- The Hon. Andrew Fahie
  Minister of Education, Culture, Sports & Youth Affairs
  British Virgin Islands

- The Hon. Roy Bodden
  Minister of Education, Human Resources & Culture
  Cayman Islands

- The Hon. Roosevelt Skerrit
  Minister of Education, Sports & Youth Affairs
  Dominica

- The Hon. Augustine John
  Minister of Education
  Grenada
- The Hon. Dr. Henry Jeffrey
  Minister of Education
  Guyana

- Mme. Myrto Celestin Saurel
  Ministre de l'Éducation nationale
  Haiti

- The Hon. Maxine Henry-Wilson
  Minister of Education, Youth & Culture
  Jamaica

- The Hon. Emely de Jongh-Elhage
  Minister of Education, Youth, Sports & Culture
  Netherlands Antilles

- The Hon. Timothy Harris
  Minister of Foreign Affairs & Education
  St. Kitts & Nevis

- The Hon. Mario Michel
  Minister of Education
  St. Lucia

- The Hon. Michael Brown
  Minister of Education, Youth & Sports
  St. Vincent & the Grenadines

- The Hon. Walter T. Sandriman
  Minister of Education & Community Development
  Suriname

- The Hon. Hazel Manning
  Minister of Education
  Trinidad & Tobago

APPENDIX 2

Rapid Appraisal Framework for HIV/AIDS and Education

The Rapid Appraisal Framework presents a set of questions that can help to assess the progress of the education sector in equipping itself to counter HIV/AIDS. The answers a user gives to these questions give some indication of the extent to which the sector has or has not mobilized itself to cope with the many situations involved in a comprehensive response by education to the epidemic.

The questions are grouped in four strategic areas:

1. *Foundation for action*: basic conditions on the grounds that they are a prerequisite to all that follows. The questions in this area deal with policy aspects, the regulatory framework, leadership, and partnerships.

2. *Assessment and information needs*: actions designed to improve understanding of the consequences of the epidemic for the sector and to generate additional knowledge and understanding. Questions are grouped under three headings: vulnerability and risk profile; impact assessment; and social assessment.

3. *Planning and implementation*: the extent to which the education sector is taking systematic steps to respond to the epidemic. Questions deal with strategic planning, costs and financial resources, the management framework, and capacity assessment.

4. *Key interventions*: purposeful action being undertaken within the education sector to respond to identified aspects of the epidemic. The principal intervention areas are curriculum,

teacher development and materials; awareness, advocacy and sensitization; counselling and testing; and health services.

The Rapid Appraisal Framework can be used at any stage of planning and implementation, but is of particular value in guiding the strategic planning process.

To complete the form, read first the question in the column headed 'Strategic Area' and then, as appropriate, tick one of the columns marked 'yes', 'no', 'action being planned', 'action in progress', or 'do not know'. Having assessed the present situation in this simple way, proceed to identify, in the right hand column, areas where possible action could be taken. For example, you may indicate that nothing is being done in a particular area, but then go on to identify some action that would help to change this situation. In areas that have already seen action, you might wish to suggest further actions that would enhance the ability of the sector to respond to the epidemic.

The Framework can help in sensitising an educator to the complexities involved in responding to the HIV/AIDS situation through one's own education system. It can also be valuable for developing a common understanding within members of a national group on what is or is not being done and what needs to be done.

Rapid appraisal framework for HIV/AIDS and education

Strategic area	Assessment				Action	
	Yes	No	Action in progress	Action being planned	Do not know	Possible Action
First strategic area Foundation for action						
Policy aspects						
Does the sector have a policy for HIV/AIDS and education?						
Has this policy been disseminated across the sector?						
Does the policy cover the entire education sector?						

Strategic area	Assessment				Action	
	Yes	No	Action in progress	Action being planned	Do not know	Possible Action
Is the policy comprehensive, covering all areas relating to HIV/AIDS and education?						
Has the education policy on HIV/AIDS been linked to the national AIDS policy?						
Is there an AIDS-in-the-workplace policy for the information and protection of the sectors workforce?						
Regulatory framework						
Has the education ministry developed codes of conduct and procedures for dealing with aspects of HIV/AIDS in staff and institutions?						
Have these been disseminated?						
Are they adequate?						
Are they being conscientiously and predictably applied						
Is the education ministry operating in accordance with legislation or international agreements?						
Leadership						
Do the political leaders in education show clear commitment to the proactive management of HIV/AIDS within the sector?						
Do senior education officials show this commitment?						
Do teachers unions and teacher leaders show this commitment?						

Strategic area	Assessment				Action	
	Yes	No	Action in progress	Action being planned	Do not know	Possible Action
Do school governing bodies and/or parent-teacher associations show this commitment?						
Are the political leaders in education well informed about what HIV/AIDS means or could mean in the sector?						
Are senior education officials well informed on this?						
Are school governing bodies and/or parent-teacher associations well informed?						
Does responsibility for HIV/AIDS action within the education ministry lie at a sufficiently senior level?						
Partnerships						
Does the education ministry involve other government agencies/ministries in its fight against HIV/AIDS?						
Does it involve the private sector?						
Does it involve non-governmental organisations?						
Does it involve faith-based organisations and the churches?						
Does it involve school governing bodies and/or parent-teacher associations?						
Do mechanisms exist that encourage partnership involvement?						

Strategic area	Assessment				Action	
	Yes	No	Action in progress	Action being planned	Do not know	Possible Action
Second strategic area Assessments and in formation needs						
Vulnerability and risk profile						
Has an assessment been made of the factors that make learners susceptible to HIV infection?						
Has an assessment been made of factors that might increase the susceptibility of teachers and educators to HIV infection?						
Have any steps been taken to deal with any of these factors?						
Are education institutions safe places for all learners and teachers (free from physical and sexual violence)?						
Do education institutions operate within a framework of strong concern for the exercise of human rights?						
Is there a policy of zero tolerance for any HIV/AIDS-related manifestation of stigma or discriminations?						
Is this policy implemented?						
Impact assessment						
Does the ministry collect information about HIV/AIDS among learners, teachers and members of its workforce?						
Does the ministry collect information on how HIV/AIDS is affecting its operations?						

Strategic area	Assessment				Action	
	Yes	No	Action in progress	Action being planned	Do not know	Possible Action
Has the ministry conducted a study assessing the impact of HIV/AIDS on the sector?						
Does the ministry intend to conduct such a study in the future?						
Is information about HIV/AIDS and education used to adjust decisions, procedures, funding, policy measures?						
Has the educational management information system (EMIS) been adjusted to incorporate HIV/AIDS perspectives and issues?						
Social assessment						
Is the ministry properly informed on the number of learners infected with HIV?						
Is the ministry adequately informed on the number of learners affected by HIV/AIDS in their families or communities?						
Is the ministry properly informed on the number of orphans in need of educational provision?						
Is the ministry well-informed on the strategies that families and communities use in responding to the physical, social and emotional needs of orphans?						
Is the ministry taking steps to improve its information in these areas?						

Strategic area	Assessment				Action	
	Yes	No	Action in progress	Action being planned	Do not know	Possible Action
Does the ministry plan to take any special measures to ensure that orphans and children made vulnerable by HIV/AIDS can exercise their right to quality education?						
Does the ministry have information on how many teachers and others in its workforce are infected with HIV?						
Is the ministry taking any special steps to respond to the needs of teachers and other members of its workforce who are infected with HIV?						
Third strategic area planning and implementation						
Strategic planning						
Is there an education sector HIV/AIDS strategic plan?						
Does the plan cover every sub-sector, from pre-primary up to university?						
Does the plan include participation by partners outside the government?						
Does the plan identify units or posts that will be responsible for plan implementation?						
Costs and financial resources						
Have costed priorities for action been developed?						
Have resources for plan implementation been provided for within the national budget for education?						

Strategic area	Assessment				Action	
	Yes	No	Action in progress	Action being planned	Do not know	Possible Action
Have efforts been made to mobilize from other sources resources for plan implementation?						
Are funds for responding to HIV/AIDS being channelled to every level of the education sector?						
Are funds for responding to HIV/AIDS being channelled to NGOs, faith-based organisations, and other partners outside of government?						
Management framework						
Has the unit that will be responsible for the implementation of the HIV/AIDS strategic plan been clearly defined and given the necessary authority?						
Does this unit have its counterparts at lower levels of the system?						
Does this unit have adequate capacity (human, financial, material resources)?						
Are any steps being taken to build the capacity of this unit through short-term and long-term training or through purpose-designed attachments?						
Is the person who heads this unit senior enough to be able to ensure that things happen?						
Capacity assessment						
Have steps been taken to make every member of the ministry workforce AIDS-competent?						

Strategic area		Assessment				Action	
	Yes	No	Action in progress	Action being planned	Do not know	Possible Action
Is training being provided to equip senior and middle level managers to respond creatively to the impacts and demands of HIV/AIDS?							
Have staff in ministry headquarters and regional/district offices been familiarised with the potential of HIV/AIDS to undermine the education system?							
Have these staff been sensitized to the need to mainstream HIV/AIDS perspectives into their routine tasks?							
Fourth strategic area Key interventions							
Curriculum, teacher development, and materials							
Does the curriculum make express provision for skills-based learning in the areas of (a) HIV/AIDS, (b) sexual and reproductive health (SRH), and (c) life-skills? (a) (b) (c)							
Is teaching in these areas conducted for all learners, from pre-primary to senior secondary?							
Is education in any of these areas a required component of the programmes of studies at post-secondary level?							
Is teaching in these areas integrated into wider skills-based health programmes?							

Strategic area	Assessment			Action		
	Yes	No	Action in progress	Action being planned	Do not know	Possible Action
Is education in any of these areas a required component of the programmes of studies at post-secondary level?						
Is teaching in these areas integrated into wider skills-based health programmes?						
Are teachers and other education personnel adequately equipped to deliver the necessary messages about HIV/AIDS and/or sexual and reproductive health?						
Are steps being taken to ensure the competence of every serving teacher for HIV preventive education?						
Are HIV/AIDS, SRH, and life-skills integral components in the curriculum for the professional preparation of all new teachers?						
Do educational institutions have the curriculum materials they need to support HIV prevention teaching activities?						
Does every teacher have access to such materials?						
Does every learner have appropriate access to such materials?						
Have steps been taken to ensure the consistency of HIV prevention messages through the sector (that is, to ensure that messages do not conflict with one another)?						

Strategic area	Assessment				Action	
	Yes	No	Action in progress	Action being planned	Do not know	Possible Action
Have efforts been made to ensure that parents and guardians are comfortable with the HIV prevention messages and materials used within the sector?						
Have efforts been made to ensure that religious leaders and faith-based organisations support the HIV prevention approach adopted by the education sector, the messages it communicates and the materials it uses?						
Is any back-up provided to schools or teachers in the area of HIV preventive education (quality assurance measures, seminars, group sessions, etc)?						
Awareness, advocacy and sensitization						
Are activities conducted to heighten among education leaders, politicians and education partners awareness of HIV and its implications for education?						
Are there any such activities for (a) learners, (b) teachers, (c) other education staff? (a) (b) (c)						
Do ministry publications carry articles or news-briefs on HIV/AIDS and education?						
Does the ministry promote the use of HIV/AIDS 'edutainment' materials on radio and television?						

Strategic area		Assessment			Action		
	Yes	No	Action in progress	Action being planned	Do not know	Possible Action	
Counselling and testing							
Do learners and educators affected or infected by HIV/AIDS have ready access to the necessary psycho-social counselling?							
Is there a policy advocating the use by learners and educators of voluntary counselling and testing (VCT)?							
Are VCT facilities readily accessible by all learners and educators?							
Do learners and educators use these facilities?							
Health services							
Have any arrangements been made with the health sector for the provision of appropriate health services in or near to educational institutions?							
Are these services friendly to young people in terms of (a) absolute confidentiality, (b) times of operation, and (c) non-judgemental atmosphere? (a) (b) (c)							
Do these centres have adequate supplies and materials?							

Note: This Rapid Appraisal Framework has been developed from the original version devised by Carol Coombe and an edited version of this produced by the Mobile Task Team, University of Natal, Durban, South Africa.

APPENDIX 3

Clearinghouses and Websites for Education and HIV/AIDS

UNESCO has established two clearinghouses dealing with education and HIV/AIDS, one at the International Institute for Educational Planning (IIEP) on the impact of HIV/AIDS on education, the other at the International Bureau of Education (IBE) on curriculum products and processes related to HIV/AIDS prevention education at primary and secondary school levels.

International Institute for Educational Planning: www.unesco.org/iiep

The IIEP HIV/AIDS Impact on Education clearinghouse web site can be consulted by going to IIEP's homepage and clicking on the clearinghouse link on the right-hand side. The site deals with both formal and non formal education systems, and presents materials coming from education ministries, researchers, NGOs, university faculties of education, management institutions, documentation centres and international agencies. The documentation on the site deals mostly with the impact of HIV/AIDS on education systems; methods for measuring impact; and best practices and measures to help curb as well as cope with the effects of the pandemic.

In practice the IIEP clearinghouse covers all of the following documents:

- policy documents related to HIV/AIDS impact on education;

- studies and research related to the planning, implementation and evaluation of HIV/AIDS education policies and programmes;
- descriptions/case studies of good practice to mitigate HIV/AIDS impact on education systems;
- Conference proceedings.

Key features of the clearinghouse include:

- hundreds of easy-to-download documents in PDF format;
- easy search facility by author, keyword, content, document title, or geographical keyword;
- abstracts for 90 per cent of the documents;
- summaries of longer documents;
- links to over 60 HIV/AIDS web sites;
- regularly updated calendar of HIV/AIDS events from around the world;
- online glossary of AIDS and education terms as well as acronyms and abbreviations.

International Bureau of Education: www.unesco.org/ibe

The IBE international clearinghouse focuses on curriculum processes and practice in education for the prevention and mitigation of HIV/AIDS. The site provides access to documents that record and analyse curriculum products and processes related to HIV/AIDS prevention education at primary and secondary school levels, with emphasis on official curricula. The role of the clearinghouse is both to disseminate and evaluate information on curriculum practice relating to HIV/AIDS education. The clearinghouse facility is directed at education specialists and other professionals working in the area of curriculum design, implementation and evaluation for the prevention and mitigation of HIV/AIDS at national, regional and international levels.

Materials handled by the clearinghouse include:

- curriculum documents (frameworks, plans, syllabi) for use in schools and teacher training institutes;
- teaching materials and teaching aids (including a range of media formats);

- studies and research related to curriculum development, implementation and evaluation;
- descriptions/case studies of good practice of HIV/AIDS curriculum related material.

Other potentially useful sites

AIDS Education Global Information System: www.aegis.org

The AIDS Education Global Information System (AEGIS) was conceived as a global informational response to the global AIDS pandemic. The web site provides large databases of new articles, information from US government sources, and more.

Education International: www.ei-ie.org/aids

The web site of Education International (EI), dedicated to school health and HIV/AIDS prevention related work. The objectives of the website are to inform, to allow access to various information, EI activities and actions related to HIV/AIDS issue and school health and HIV/AIDS prevention in particular. The website reports on various actions and activities undertaken by EI and its partners (WHO, EDC, CDC, UNICEF, UNESCO and UNAIDS) since 1995.

Family Health International: www.fhi.org

The Family Health International (FHI) website provides information on FHI programs in developing countries to prevent the spread of HIV/AIDS and sexually transmitted diseases and improve care for people with HIV/AIDS. Through its YouthNet programme, FHI gives information on its work to prevent HIV/AIDS and improve the reproductive health of young people aged 10 to 24 years.

Health Economics and HIV/AIDS Research Division: www.und.ac.za/und/heard

Information on publications, policy developments, and impacts of HIV/AIDS on socio-economic development. AIDS briefs and AIDS toolkits can be downloaded from the site.

HIV InSite. www.hivinsite.org

Developed by the Center for HIV Information (CHI) at the University of California San Francisco (UCSF), HIV InSite's mission is to be a source for comprehensive, in-depth HIV/AIDS information and knowledge.

Low cost teaching aids: www.talc.org

Provides information on low-cost teaching and other materials for HIV/AIDS and how to access these.

Orphans and vulnerable children

www.displacedchildrenandorphansfund.org/
www.childrensaidsfund.org/cmdb/index.htm
www.orphans.fxb.org

UNAIDS: www.unaids.org

The site of the joint United Nations Programme on HIV/AIDS, providing wide-ranging global, regional and country level epidemiological information on the progress of the epidemic. The site also provides case studies on best practice. The annual Update on the AIDS epidemic can be downloaded from this site.

UNESCO: www.unesco.org

The main UNESCO site with links to UNESCO publications and a wide range of education documents. UNESCO's strategy for HIV/AIDS preventive education, the Inter-Agency Task Team's Education and HIV/AIDS. A strategic approach, and the annual EFA global monitoring report can be downloaded from this site.

UNFPA: www.unfpa.org

Deals with sexual and reproductive health. The annual publication State of the world's population and a series of HIV prevention briefs can be downloaded from the site.

UNICEF: www.unicef.org

The site of UNICEF providing articles and press releases on HIV/
AIDS in relation to children and young people, as well as country-
by-country general statistical information on children and young
people. The annual report *State of the world's children* can be
downloaded from the site.

World Bank: www.worldbank.org

The central World Bank site, with links to World Bank publications,
country profiles, and documents in the HIV/AIDS and Education
series, including A window of hope and A sourcebook of HIV/AIDS
prevention programs.

INDEX

Printed in the United States
21742LVS00002B/1-44